Psychosocial Group Work with Vulnerable Children

T0372823

Psychosocial Group Work with Vulnerable Children presents a simple, accessible and preventative approach to psychotherapeutic interventions.

The authors explore how this form of group work can strengthen resilience and prevent an increase in antisocial behavioural tendencies among children. Based on a process of shared meaning communication, the book explains how professionals can help children to engage in in-group creative play and allow them to experience their self in relation to others. Castrechini-Franieck (also known as 'Maria Leticia Castrechini Fernandes Franieck') and Bittner draw on their experiences of working with children in groups, supplemented with therapeutic elements from Gestalt therapy and ontological psychoanalysis. This approach helps children to achieve a stable state of emotional well-being while improving their behaviour at school, along with their social skills.

Psychosocial Group Work with Vulnerable Children will be a key reading for psychotherapists and other professionals working with vulnerable children including psychologists, psychiatrists and social workers.

Maria Leticia Castrechini Fernandes Franieck, PhD, is a registered Chartered Counselling Psychologist in the UK, an in-training Group Analyst with the Seminar für Gruppenanalyse Zürich, and a licensed psychoanalytic Psychotherapist and Supervisor in Germany. Working with highly vulnerable populations is central to her clinical practice, and her studies were funded by the International Psychoanalytical Association.

Niko Bittner is a qualified pedagogue and Gestalt therapist, as well as a systemic trainer and coach. He works in youth social work and is a seminar leader at the Odenwald Institute, Germany, where he trains conflict coaches, among other things.

The Forensic Psychotherapy Monograph Series

The Official Publication Series of the International Association for Forensic Psychotherapy
Series Editor: Professor Brett Kahr

Disabling Perversions: Forensic Psychotherapy with People with Intellectual Disabilities
Alan Corbett

Sexual Abuse and the Sexual Offender: Common Man or Monster?
Barry Maletzky

Psychotherapy with Male Survivors of Sexual Abuse: The Invisible Men
Alan Corbett

Consulting to Chaos: An Approach to Patient-Centred Reflective Practice
Edited by John Gordon, Gabriel Kirtchuk, Maggie McAlister, and David Reiss

Sadism: Psychoanalytic Developmental Perspectives
Edited by Amita Sehgal

The End of the Sentence: Psychotherapy with Female Offenders
Edited by Pamela Windham Stewart and Jessica Collier

Communicating with Vulnerable Patients: A Novel Psychological Approach
Maria Leticia Castrechini Fernandes Franieck

Psychosocial Group Work with Vulnerable Children: Eclectic Group Conductors and Creative Play
Maria Leticia Castrechini Fernandes Franieck & Niko Bittner

For further information about this series please visit https://www.routledge.com/
The-Forensic-Psychotherapy-Monograph-Series/book-series/KARNFPM

Psychosocial Group Work with Vulnerable Children

Eclectic Group Conductors and Creative Play

Maria Leticia
Castrechini Fernandes Franieck
and Niko Bittner

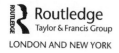

Routledge
Taylor & Francis Group
LONDON AND NEW YORK

Designed cover image: © Maria Leticia Castrechini Fernandes Franieck

First published 2025
by Routledge
4 Park Square, Milton Park, Abingdon, Oxon OX14 4RN

and by Routledge
605 Third Avenue, New York, NY 10158

Routledge is an imprint of the Taylor & Francis Group, an informa business

Psychosoziale Gruppenarbeit mit benachteiligten Kindern; Paarleitung und kreatives Spiel

by Maria Leticia Castrechini Fernandes Franieck and Niko Bittner, edition: 1

Copyright © Der/die Herausgeber bzw. der/die Autor(en), exklusiv lizenziert an Springer Fachmedien Wiesbaden GmbH, ein Teil von Springer Nature, 2023 *

This edition has been translated and published under licence from

Springer Fachmedien Wiesbaden GmbH, part of Springer Nature.

Springer Fachmedien Wiesbaden GmbH, part of Springer Nature takes no responsibility and shall not be made liable for the accuracy of the translation.

British Library Cataloguing-in-Publication Data
A catalogue record for this book is available from the British Library

ISBN: 978-1-032-73946-5 (hbk)
ISBN: 978-1-032-73945-8 (pbk)
ISBN: 978-1-003-46685-7 (ebk)

DOI: 10.4324/9781003466857

Typeset in Times New Roman
by Taylor & Francis Books

To all vulnerable children and young people who allowed me to come into contact with them, without which I could not have written this book. I have learnt a lot from each of you. Thanks!

To my colleague Niko Bittner, for being my loyal colleague throughout this emotional work and above all for supporting me in rediscovering the playfulness and creativity inside of me, so I could find my way! — Maria Leticia Castrechini Fernandes Franieck

To all who have challenged me on my career path involving children and youths, and to those who continue to do so. To my family, my two sons, who were among these children and young people, and to my wife and her patient companionship.

To my colleague Leticia, to her conviction in this book, her incredible perseverance — without her, this would not really have been possible. — Niko Bittner

Contents

List of illustrations   ix
Forensic Psychotherapy Monograph Series: Series editor's
foreword   x
German foreword: 'Together We Are Strong!' – T-WAS   xv
Preface   xvii
Acknowledgements   xviii

Introduction   1

PART I
Conceptual source of inspiration   5

1 The interplay between antisocial tendencies and aggression   7

2 Relating Gestalt therapy to ontological psychoanalysis   16

3 Running a group in partnership: What does this mean?   24

PART 2
Together We Are Strong (T-WAS)   33

4 The challenges behind the scenes   35

5 'Eclectic group conductors'   40

6 Settings   50

7 Creative play   58

8 Three different children's groups   88

9 Direct challenges from children to eclectic group conductors 100

10 Reflections on T-WAS (Together We Are Strong) 119

Index 126

Illustrations

Figures

5.1 Eclectic group conductors reference points. 42
5.2 Eclectic group conductors roles. 43
5.3 Niko glued. 46
6.1 Approach-pillars. 51
7.1 Playing court. 66
7.2 Rubber chicken. 70
8.1 Group overview. 89
8.2 Printer room. 92
8.3 Cover of the photo book. 94
10.1 Classification. 122

Tables

I.1 Short films produced for the presentation at the 51st Congress
of the International Psychoanalytic Association in London, UK 3
7.1 Short films produced during the COVID-19 pandemic (first and
second waves) 83

Forensic Psychotherapy Monograph Series: Series editor's foreword

In 1801, the English judiciary condemned a 13-year-old boy to death and then hanged him on the gallows at Tyburn, in the heart of London. But what crime had he committed? Apparently, this young lad had stolen merely a spoon (Westwick 1940). Tragically, during the early nineteenth century, such an infraction could actually result in capital punishment.

Throughout much of human history, our ancestors have performed rather poorly when responding to acts of violence. In most cases, our predecessors will either have *ignored* murderousness, as in the case of Graeco-Roman infanticide, which occurred so regularly in the ancient world that it acquired an almost normative status (deMause 1974; Kahr 1994); or they will have *punished* destructive behaviours with retaliatory sadism, a form of unconscious identification with the aggressor. Any history of criminology will readily reveal the cruel punishments inflicted upon prisoners throughout the ages, ranging from beatings and stockades, to more severe forms of torture, culminating in eviscerations, lynchings, beheadings and electrocutions (e.g., Kahr 2020b).

Only during the last 100 years have we begun to develop the capacity to respond more intelligently and more humanely to dangerousness and destruction. Since the advent of psychoanalysis, we now have access to a much deeper understanding of both the aetiology of aggressive acts and their treatment; and nowadays, we need no longer ignore criminals or abuse them – instead, we can offer forensic psychotherapeutic interventions with compassion and containment, as well as conduct research which can help to prevent future acts of violence. By *treating* aggressive patients, rather than by *punishing* them, forward-thinking mental health practitioners now possess the ability to draw upon the new discipline of forensic psychotherapy, designed to understand the causes of violence, in order to help rehumanise the dehumanised.

The discipline of forensic psychotherapy can trace its origins to the very early days of psychoanalysis. On 6 February 1907, at a meeting of the Wiener Psychoanalytische Vereinigung (Vienna Psycho-Analytical Society), Professor Sigmund Freud bemoaned the often horrible treatment of mentally ill offenders. According to Herr Otto Rank, Freud's secretary at the time, the founder of psychoanalysis expressed his sorrow at the 'unsinnige Behandlung dieser Leute' (quoted in Rank 1907a, p. 101), which translates as the 'nonsensical treatment of these people' (quoted in Rank 1907b, p. 108).

Subsequently, many of the early psychoanalytical practitioners preoccupied themselves with forensic topics. Dr Hanns Sachs, himself a trained lawyer, and the Princesse Marie Bonaparte, a noted French aristocrat, spoke fiercely against capital punishment. Sachs, one of the first members of Freud's inner circle, regarded the death penalty for offenders as an example of group sadism (Moellenhoff 1966); while Bonaparte (1927), who had studied various murderers throughout her career, actually campaigned to free the convicted killer Caryl Chessman, during his sentence on Death Row at the California State Prison in San Quentin (Bertin 1982).

Some years later, Mrs Melanie Klein (1932a), the Austrian-born, British-based clinician, concluded her first book, the landmark text *Die Psycho-analyse des Kindes* – known in English as *The Psycho-Analysis of Children* (Klein 1932b) – with a truly memorable clarion call. Mrs Klein noted that acts of criminality stem invariably from disturbances in childhood, and that if young people could receive psychoanalytical treatment at an early age, then much cruelty would be prevented in later years. As she argued, 'If every child who shows disturbances that are at all severe were to be analysed in good time, a great number of these people who later end up in prisons or lunatic asylums, or who go completely to pieces, would be saved from such a fate and be able to develop a normal life' (Klein 1932b, p. 374).[1]

Shortly after the publication of Klein's transformative book, Atwell Westwick, a Judge of the Superior Court of Santa Barbara, California, published a little-known, though highly inspiring, article on 'Criminology and psychoanalysis' in *The Psychoanalytic Quarterly*. Westwick may well be the first judge to have committed himself in print to the value of psychoanalysis in the study of criminality, arguing that punishment of the forensic patient remains, in fact, a sheer waste of time. With passion, Judge Westwick (1940, p. 281) queried, 'Can we not, in our well nigh hopeless and overwhelming struggle with the problems of delinquency and crime, profit by medical experience with the problems of health and disease? Will we not, eventually, terminate the senseless policy of sitting idly by until misbehavior occurs, often with irreparable damage, then dumping the delinquent into the juvenile court or reformatory and dumping the criminal into prison?' Westwick noted that we should, instead, train judges, probation officers, social workers, as well as teachers and parents, in the precepts of psychoanalysis, in order to arrive at a more sensitive, non-punitive understanding of the nature of criminality. As Westwick (1940, p. 281) opined, 'When we shall have succeeded in committing society to such a program, when we see it launched definitely upon the venture, as in time it surely will be – then shall we have erected an appropriate memorial to Sigmund Freud'.

Although the roots of forensic psychotherapy stem back to the early years of the twentieth century (e.g., Kahr 2018; 2022), the discipline only became constellated more formally in the 1980s and 1990s, due, in large measure, to the pioneering work of the esteemed forensic psychiatrist and forensic psychotherapist, Dr Estela Valentina Welldon (1988; 1996; 2002; 2011; 2015), and many of her colleagues, and, thankfully, the profession now boasts a much more robust foundation, with training courses available for young mental health workers in the UK and beyond. Since the inauguration of the Diploma in Forensic Psychotherapy, created by Dr Welldon, hosted by the Portman Clinic in London, and sponsored by the British Postgraduate Medical Federation of the University of London, with the support and encouragement of its leader, Professor Sir Michael Peckham (Kahr 2021), students can now seek further instruction in the psychodynamic treatment of patients who act out in a dangerous and illegal manner. Dr Welldon – subsequently Professor Welldon – created not only the world's first training programme in forensic psychotherapy, but she also launched the International Association for Forensic Psychotherapy in 1991, and hosted its first conference in 1992 at St. Bartholomew's Hospital in London. This passionate and devoted organisation has certainly helped to develop the field globally.

Back in 1997, at the kind invitation of Mr Cesare Sacerdoti, the owner of H. Karnac (Books) at that time, I had the privilege of commissioning a host of titles for a new book series, designed to promote this growing branch of forensic psychological assessment, treatment and prevention; and the very first titles appeared several years later (Bloom 2001; Kahr 2001; Saunders 2001). Over time, this Forensic Psychotherapy Monograph Series, now published by Routledge, part of the Taylor and Francis Group, has endeavoured to produce a regular stream of high-quality titles, written by leading members of the profession, who share their expertise in a concise and practice-orientated fashion. We trust that this collection of books, which, in 2022, became the official monograph series of the International Association for Forensic Psychotherapy, will help to consolidate and to disseminate the knowledge and experience that we have already acquired, and will also provide more creative pathways in the decades to come.

Happily, our growing field of forensic psychotherapy boasts many creative and productive colleagues, not least, Dr Maria Leticia Castrechini Fernandes Franieck, an esteemed psychologist and group psychoanalyst, who has already published a very important book on *Communicating with Vulnerable Patients: A Novel Psychological Approach*, as part of the Forensic Psychotherapy Monograph Series (Castrechini-Franieck, 2022), in which she drew upon her vast experience of working with traumatised patients in detention centres and in psychiatric hospitals.

In her newest book, *Psychosocial Group Work with Deprived Children: Eclectic Group Conductors and Creative Play*, written in collaboration with her longstanding colleague Niko Bittner, the author expands upon her vital work, now known as T-WAS – an acronym for her transformative project, 'Together We Are Strong' – designed to help deprived refugee youngsters. By intervening early, our colleagues have made a very important contribution not only to the healing of troubled boys and girls but, also, to assisting with the prevention of criminal offences in years to come (cf. Kahr 2004; 2020a; 2020b).

Across the chapters herein, Castrechini-Franieck and Bittner describe their joint work with no fewer than 70 children and adolescents. One cannot but be deeply moved by the warm-hearted, empathic, detailed and hope-enhancing manner in which these colleagues have facilitated such important, transformative work. I remain hopeful – indeed, confident – that this book will help to inspire future generations of forensic mental health practitioners and many other people besides.

As the new millennium begins to unfold, we now have an opportunity for psychotherapeutically inclined forensic mental health professionals to work in close conjunction with child psychologists and with infant mental health specialists so that the problems of violence can be tackled not only retrospectively but, also, preventatively. With the growth of the field of forensic psychotherapy, we at last have reason to be optimistic that serious criminality can be forestalled and perhaps, one day, even eradicated.

Professor Brett Kahr
Series Editor
Forensic Psychotherapy Monograph Series
International Association for Forensic Psychotherapy
Copyright © 2025, by Professor Brett Kahr.
Please do not quote without the permission of the author.

Note

1 The original German phrase reads: 'Würde jedes Kind, das ernstere Störungen zeigt, rechtzeitig der Analyse unterzogen, dann könnte wohl ein großer Teil jener Menschen, die andernfalls in Gefängnissen und Irrenhäusern landen oder sonst völlig scheitern, vor diesem Schicksal bewahrt bleiben und sich zu normalen Menschen entwickeln' (Klein 1932a, p. 293).

References

Bertin, C., 1982. *La Dernière Bonaparte*. Paris: Librairie Académique Perrin.

Bloom, S.L., ed., 2001. *Violence: A Public Health Menace and a Public Health Approach*. London: H. Karnac (Books).

Bonaparte, M., 1927. Le cas de Madame Lefebvre. *Revue Française de Psychanalyse*, 1, 149–198.

deMause, L., 1974. The Evolution of Childhood. In Lloyd deMause (Ed.). *The History of Childhood*, pp. 1–73. New York: Psychohistory Press.

Castrechini-Franieck, L., 2022. *Communicating with Vulnerable Patients: A Novel Psychological Approach*. London, Abingdon: Routledge / Taylor and Francis Group.

Kahr, B., 1994. The historical foundations of ritual abuse: An excavation of ancient infanticide. In V. Sinason (ed.), *Treating Survivors of Satanist Abuse*. London: Routledge, 45–56.

Kahr, B., ed., 2001. *Forensic Psychotherapy and Psychopathology: Winnicottian Perspectives*. London: H. Karnac (Books).

Kahr, B. 2004. Juvenile paedophilia: The psychodynamics of an adolescent. In C.W. Socarides and L.R. Loeb (eds.), *The Mind of the Paedophile: Psychoanalytic Perspectives*. London: H. Karnac (Books), 95–119.

Kahr, B., 2018. 'No intolerable persons' or 'lewd pregnant women': Towards a history of forensic psychoanalysis. In B. Kahr (ed.), *New Horizons in Forensic Psychotherapy: Exploring the Work of Estela V. Welldon*. London: H. Karnac (Books), 17–87.

Kahr, B., 2020a. *Bombs in the Consulting Room: Surviving Psychological Shrapnel*. London, Abingdon: Routledge / Taylor and Francis Group.

Kahr, B., 2020b. *Dangerous Lunatics: Trauma, Criminality, and Forensic Psychotherapy*. London: Confer Books.

Kahr, B., 2021. Professor Sir Michael Peckham: A memorial tribute. *International Journal of Forensic Psychotherapy*, 3, 163–165.

Kahr, B., 2022. 'Let the great axe fall': From Ancient Babylonian torture to modern forensic psychotherapy: Freud, Welldon, and the humanisation of criminality. *International Journal of Forensic Psychotherapy*, 4, 89–118.

Klein, M., 1932a. *Die Psychoanalyse des Kindes*. Vienna: Internationaler Psychoanalytischer Verlag.

Klein, M., 1932b. *The Psycho-Analysis of Children*. A. Strachey (transl.). London: Hogarth Press and the Institute of Psycho-Analysis.

Moellenhoff, F., 1966. Hanns Sachs. 1881–1947: The creative unconscious. In F. Alexander, S. Eisenstein and M. Grotjahn (eds.), *Psychoanalytic Pioneers*. New York: Basic Books, 180–199.

Rank, O., ed., 1907a. Vortragsabend: Am 6. Februar 1907. In H. Nunberg and E. Federn (eds.) (1976), *Protokolle der Wiener Psychoanalytischen Vereinigung: Band I. 1906–1908*. Frankfurt am Main: S. Fischer Verlag, 97–104.

Rank, O., ed., 1907b. Scientific meeting on February 6, 1907. In H. Nunberg and E. Federn (eds.) (1962), *Minutes of the Vienna Psychoanalytic Society. Volume 1: 1906–1908*. M. Nunberg (transl.). New York: International Universities Press, 103–110.

Saunders, J.W., ed., 2001. *Life Within Hidden Walls: Psychotherapy in Prisons*. London: H. Karnac (Books).

Welldon, E.V., 1988. *Mother, Madonna, Whore: The Idealization and Denigration of Motherhood*. London: Free Association Books.

Welldon, E.V., 1996. Contrasts in male and female sexual perversions. In C. Cordess and M. Cox (eds.), *Forensic Psychotherapy: Crime, Psychodynamics and the Offender Patient*. Volume 2: *Mainly Practice*. London: Jessica Kingsley Publishers, 273–289.

Welldon, E.V., 2002. *Sadomasochism*. Duxford, Cambridge: Icon Books.

Welldon, E.V., 2011. *Playing with Dynamite: A Personal Approach to the Psychoanalytic Understanding of Perversions, Violence, and Criminality*. London: Karnac Books.

Welldon, E.V., 2015. Forensic psychotherapy. *Psychoanalytic Psychotherapy*, 29, 211–227.

Westwick, A., 1940. Criminology and psychoanalysis. *Psychoanalytic Quarterly*, 9, 269–282.

German foreword: 'Together We Are Strong!' – T-WAS

It is both a great honour and pleasure for me to be able to introduce the impressive *Psychosocial Group Work with Vulnerable Children* by Niko Bittner and Maria Leticia Castrechini Fernandes Franieck. These are several open group projects, with multi-traumatised refugee children, supported over a range of different time periods under a shared leadership. 'Together We Are Strong!' is the motto, as well as the approach of Bittner and Castrechini-Franieck's work, and can serve as such for the continuously growing community of those who work with children's and young people's groups, in a wide variety of professional contexts. 'T-WAS – Together We Are Strong!' already focuses in its title on two significant effective powers of groups: the experience of cohesion and belonging, and also implicitly its destructive antipodes of fragmentation and being excluded. According to the authors, their preventive work aims at strengthening the resilience of the children in their care and is aimed at preventing the increase of antisocial and destructive-aggressive behavioural tendencies of this special clientele. The authors consistently rely on the developmental effect of experience-based group processes in the here and now, on relationship-focused guidance and on the possibility of free play. Supplemented by their model of 'eclectic group conductors' (chapter 5), the concept presented by Bittner and Castrechini-Franieck is characterised by these three points of reference as a further, enriching facet of genuinely group-analytical work with children and adolescents, as it is fanned out in the anthology *Gruppenanalytisch arbeiten mit Kindern und Jugendlichen – Impulse für eine kreative und vielfältige Praxis* (*Working Group-Analytically with Children and Adolescents – Impulses for a Creative and Diverse Practice*) recently published by Stumptner (2022) as an expression of a 'lived diversity' of group-analytical work (p. 12). Also, and especially through the cultivation of their eclectic group conductors both as a team of authors and in the model of equal pair leadership – Bittner and Castrechini-Franieck expand the view of the diverse 'landscapes of group analysis with children and adolescents' (ibid. p. 11) with another valuable perspective. Bittner, a qualified pedagogue and Gestalt therapist, coming from youth social work, and Castrechini-Franieck, a doctor of psychology and licensed psychodynamic psychotherapist, associated with ontological psycho-analysis and with great experience with particularly vulnerable patient groups, for example from the field of forensic psychiatry, use the different roots of their professional socialisation for the very special balancing act of 'shared meaning communication' (Castrechini-Franieck and Bittner, 2022), which, in addition to all the basic commonalities, also shows curiosity and appreciative attention to the respective different, sometimes seemingly unfamiliar 'others'. Particularly impressive is the openness with which Leticia and Niko consciously bring in their conceivably different personal biographies (chapter 4) as 'challenges behind the scenes' that always resonate in the work, partly reflected together, partly supervised separately, and make them useful for group analysis. In this way, despite all their differences, the two discover 'astonishing commonalities' ranging from self-experienced exclusion and foreignness to deprivation and violence. Both have 'overcome painful experiences and constructively processed them in order to then integrate them into their career choices'. This is where the authors see 'the source of their desire to work with vulnerable children'. Chapter 8 describes this work through touching case vignettes of three different groups of children in different shared housing for refugees. We witness the particular challenge of working with this clientele and responding appropriately to their enormous insecurity, fear and mistrust. The authors talk about the initial 'chaos', the inability to grasp and articulate thoughts, and the impotent attempts of traumatised children to counter fears of loss with aggression. The authors contrast this with the security of a stable, protected framework, community experiences based on sport and play and, above all, the offer of reliable and authentic relationship experiences, which also include coping with farewells, anger and grief together. Especially in this chapter, it becomes noticeable how significant love is for constructive development and healing processes, and also that it alone is not enough.

Hans Georg Lehle
Ulm, 12 January 2023

References

Castrechini-Franieck, L., and Bittner, N., 2022. T-WAS: Together We Are Strong. In L. Castrechini-Franieck (ed.), *Communication with Vulnerable Patients: A Novel Psychological Approach*. London: Routledge, 155–185.

Stumptner, K., ed., 2022. *Gruppenanalytisch arbeiten mit Kindern und Jugendlichen. Impulse für eine kreative und vielfältige Praxis*. Göttingen: Vandenhoeck & Ruprecht.

Preface

How did the idea of this book come about? After the group sessions, there was a great need on our part for exchange, and we started to keep a regular record of the sessions. This led more and more to the idea of creating a book. A book that could not only reveal the challenges faced whilst leading a group of vulnerable children (including feasible failures on our part), but one that could also reveal the courage to try out new things every time when a daunting challenge was posed to the role shared by the two group leaders. The purpose of this book is to pass on the experiences we have had, as we think that they might be of some value. Along these lines, we would like to encourage and inspire more professionals who work with children to do the same. After all, the number of vulnerable children in the world is sadly not small. Indeed, from our experience, the children's responses to our approach involved great engagement and openness. A total of more than 70 children have been involved in our group work and most of them have achieved a balanced emotional well-being while improving their behaviour at school and social skills.

Acknowledgements

We wish to acknowledge our gratitude to the international religious organisation that sponsored our group work, as well as granting permission for us to report on the group work for the purposes of this book, on the understanding that the names would remain anonymous.

We owe thanks to all our colleagues who supported our work over three years in the three different shared housing for refugees, above all for their valuable help during the COVID-19 pandemic. Thanks also to those who provided us with their written appreciation and/or criticisms of this book.

We also extend our warmest appreciation to Roosevelt Smerke Cassorla, Michael Günter, Hans Lehle and Monika Mohl for their remarkable contributions while writing this book, as well as to Heather McClelland for smoothing out our English.

Our gratitude to all the vulnerable children and young people we had the pleasure of meeting in the course of our group work was expressed in the dedication.

For the permission to reproduce material that has already appeared in print, thanks are due to Taylor & Francis Group.

Introduction

The aim of this book is, on the one hand, to describe the experience of the authors in developing and finding increasingly effective ways of engaging with children at risk in the context of group work. On the other hand, it is intended to stimulate reflection on how personal differences (between the group leaders) can be confidently handled and jointly managed. In time, this can be integrated into an innovative form of group leadership.

The approach presented in this book – 'Together We Are Strong' or T-WAS – is a variation of the 'Transient Interactive Communication Approach' or TICA (Castrechini-Franieck 2022) and has a preventive rather than therapeutic character in working with vulnerable children.

From TICA to T-WAS

TICA (Castrechini-Franieck 2022) is an approach developed for work with adults (in individual or group-work settings) to facilitate the communication process with vulnerable/at-risk patients, suffering mostly from personality disorders and trauma. It is grounded in the principles of experience of 'mutuality' from Winnicott (1992/1987; 2018) or 'attunement' from Stern (2000/1995), and the ability of 'maternal reverie', as well as the 'container-contained model' from Bion (1959; 1984a; 1984b). Further details on these principles are provided in chapter 2. TICA uses an external/transitional object (cartoons, films, 'timeline', 'feelings wheel', etc.) as a means of creating a playful/transitional space (Winnicott 1953) between the therapist and patients, whilst offering representations for their emotional experiences (Bion 1965) through the creation of 'shared meaning communication'.

'Shared meaning communication' means the ability to embrace the perspectives of others to the extent that one can understand them, even if one does not agree with them – the basic pillar of TICA. According to Castrechini-Franieck (2022, pp. 24–35), due to the peculiar psychological features of the vulnerable/at-risk adult patients, the work should not be based on object relations, but rather on transitional objects. To put it another way, emotional communication between patient and practitioner is better facilitated through an external object than through personal interaction.

DOI: 10.4324/9781003466857-1

T-WAS, by contrast, is a preventive group work with vulnerable children against the increase of antisocial behavioural tendencies and is focused on strengthening resilience. This can be achieved through the creation of 'shared meaning communication'. In particular, shared meaning communication in T-WAS is achieved by helping children to engage in creative group play which enables them to experience themselves in relation to others, in line with the concept of ego-relatedness coined by (Winnicott, 1958). In simple terms, T-WAS is a search for new relationship experiences for children through play. According to Abram (2008, p. 1208), 'only through playing can the self be continually discovered and thus strengthened'. Hence, the two core pillars of T-WAS are: 1) the group conductors as referred to by Foulkes and Foulkes (1990) or the 'eclectic group conductors', as introduced by Castrechini-Franieck and Bittner (2022), and 2) creative play. The former can be understood as a novel means by which new experiences of family-like communication and also relevant experiences with parental representations can be offered (details in chapter 5). The latter was adopted by the authors to create a common (symbolic) language to support the communication among the group members whilst creating a playful/transitional space – similarly to TICA. The features of the creative play will be explained in more detail in chapter 7. In the German version of this book, the term 'eclectic group conductor' was replaced with the German term '*interdisziplinäre Paarleitung*'.

The authors communicate, crucially, the necessity for an experiential approach to the group work with vulnerable children. To this end, the book is divided into two parts. Part 1 focuses on conceptual sources of inspiration and includes three chapters. Chapter 1 presents the interplay among the ideas of 'antisocial tendency' from Winnicott et al. (2012/1984) and the positive facet of aggression and relates them to Foulkes and Foulkes' (1990) group matrix' concept – the starting point of T-WAS. Chapter 2 explains how the Gestalt therapeutic way of thinking could be particularly related to the onto-logical-psychoanalytic understanding to underpin T-WAS. Chapter 3 lays the groundwork for the conceptualisation of the novel concept of 'eclectic group conductors' through an overview and discussion of the contentious theoretical debate about the roles of the group leader, the co-leader/co-therapist and the pair of leaders within group work. Part 2 is focused on T-WAS itself and consists of six additional chapters. Chapter 4 reveals how, behind the scenes, the authors struggled to overcome daunting challenges posed by their personal differences, which might possibly affect the understanding and the way in which group work with vulnerable children is conducted. Chapter 5 introduces the concept of 'eclectic group conductor' in detail. Chapter 6 outlines the structural features of T-WAS. In chapter 7, the authors present their methods of creative play, with detailed practice notes on understanding guidance, including their strategy to overcome hardships brought about by the COVID-19 pandemic. Chapter 8 summarises the development and dynamics of the children's groups at three different shared housing sites for refugees and relates them to each other. In chapter 9, challenging situations in the group (i.e., the occurrence of riots/rebellion) are openly presented via full transcriptions and are further discussed, with a focus on how the 'eclectic group conductors' dealt with them.

Finally, chapter 10 discusses the outcomes and limitations of T-WAS, and further introduces the perspectives of other professionals about it.

Some observations on T-WAS

In the summer of 2019, T-WAS was presented as a community work project at the 51st Congress of the International Psychoanalytic Association in London, UK, under the title 'Mama! Papa! Where are you? Are you still there? What's wrong with you?'

Table 1.1 Short films produced for the presentation at the 51st Congress of the International Psychoanalytic Association in London, UK

Film	Plot summary	YouTube link
1.'The Beginning'	The authors chat about: how they met, what their previous expectations of the collaborative work were, and how they overcame the daunting challenges of setting up the T-WAS group. One can sense how they easily deal with their amazing diversity.	https://youtu.be/NFWki0OhUb0
2.'Roles & Conflicts'	The authors chat about their role as a pair of group conductors, who embody different representations, e.g., male/ female, father/mother, native/ foreigner. They make it clear how they deal with the interplay of their personal differences and put them into action in conflicts within and outside the group.	https://youtu.be/aAAEkIfIPTM
3.'Conflict & the Eclectic Pair Conductors'	This film is a sequel to the film 'Roles & Conflicts'. The authors talk about another intense conflict situation in the group. They explain how they experienced the effectiveness of their role as eclectic pair conductors and how that had an integrating effect on the children.	https://youtu.be/wSawflUd4Vs

Source: From Appendix 8.1, pp. 184–185, *Communicating with Vulnerable Patients: A Novel Psychological Approach*, by Maria Leticia Castrechini Fernandes Franieck, © 2023 Imprint. Published by Routledge with permission from Taylor and Francis Group.

Among other things, three explanatory videos about the development of the work with T-WAS were presented at the congress. In these videos, the authors chatted about how they met, how their idea of 'eclectic group conductors' came about, and how they overcame the challenges of creating a new approach to group work with vulnerable children. Readers will find Table I.1 summarising each video, including their respective YouTube links and QR codes.

In summer 2023, T-WAS was presented as a project under the theme 'promotion and prevention in community context' at the 18th World Congress for the World Association for Infant Mental Health in Dublin, Ireland, under the title '"Together We Are Strong" to avoid an increase in antisocial behavioural tendencies in vulnerable children'.

References

Abram, J., 2008. Donald Woods Winnicott (1896–1971): A brief introduction. *The International Journal of Psychoanalysis*, 89 (6), 1189–1217.

Bion, W.R., 1959. Attacks on linking. *The International Journal of Psychoanalysis*, 40, 308–315.

Bion, W.R., 1965. *Transformations: Change from Learning to Growth*. London: William Heinemann Medical Books.

Bion, W.R., 1984a. *Attention & Interpretation*. London: Maresfield Reprints.

Bion, W.R., 1984b. *Learning from Experience*. London: Maresfield.

Castrechini-Franieck, L., ed., 2022. *Communication with Vulnerable Patients: A Novel Psychological Approach*. London: Routledge.

Castrechini-Franieck, L., and Bittner, N., 2022. T-WAS: Together We Are Strong. In L. Castrechini-Franieck (ed.), *Communication with Vulnerable Patients: A Novel Psychological Approach*. London: Routledge, 155–185.

Foulkes, S.H., and Foulkes, E., 1990. *Selected Papers of S.H. Foulkes: Psychoanalysis and Group Analysis*. Edited and with a brief biography by E. Foulkes. London: Karnac Books.

Stern, D.N., 2000/1995. *The Motherhood Constellation: A Unified View of Parent-Infant Psychotherapy*. New York: Basic Books.

Winnicott, D.W., 1953. Transitional objects and transitional phenomena: A study of the first not-me possession. *International Journal of Psycho-Analysis*, 34, 89–97.

Winnicott, D.W., 1958. The capacity to be alone. *International Journal of Psycho-Analysis*, 39, 416–420.

Winnicott, D.W., 1992/1987. Communication between infant and mother, mother and infant, compared and contrasted. In D.W. Winnicott, *et al.*, eds., *Babies and Their Mothers*. Reading, MA, Wokingham: Addison-Wesley, 89–104.

Winnicott, D.W., *et al.*, eds., 2012/1984. *Deprivation and Delinquency*. Abingdon: Routledge.

Winnicott, D.W., 2018. The mother-infant experience of mutuality. In *Psycho-Analytic Explorations*. London: Routledge, 251–260.

Part I

Conceptual source of inspiration

The interplay between antisocial tendencies and aggression

In 2017, the authors met at an event. At that time, Castrechini-Franieck was working as a psychologist for an international religious organisation with traumatised refugees in their accommodation, as well for the Ministry of Justice in a forensic setting with incarcerated offenders awaiting trial. Bittner was working as a social pedagogue at a school and in addition as a freelance trainer of self-defence. During their chat, based on their personal biographies (see chapter 4), they noticed that both of them have similar concerns about an increase in antisocial tendencies (Winnicott et al. 2012/1984) among vulnerable children who have experienced great loss during their development (Castrechini-Franieck and Bittner 2022, pp. 159–160). From this moment on, they started thinking about feasible preventive group work with vulnerable children. However, both authors come from different theoretical backgrounds, Castrechini-Franieck from ontological psychoanalysis (Ogden 2019), Bittner from Gestalt therapy, with an emphasis on 'creative aggression' (Bach and Goldberg 1976; Perls et al. 1994). Their initial aim was to set the path for 'shared meaning communication' (Castrechini-Franieck 2022, p. 29), i.e., to develop a common conceptual understanding of: antisocial tendencies, aggression as a prism, and group formation – T-WAS's starting point.

1 Antisocial tendency as referred to by Winnicott

Winnicott et al. (2012/1984, pp. 73–85) distinguished between antisocial tendency and antisocial acts/behaviours or delinquency. It is true that aggression is a feature of both. Nonetheless, empathy and guilt are emotional responses seldom present in antisocial acts/behaviours or delinquency. As a matter of fact, both stem from the same root – deprivation triggered by environmental failure. Whilst the latter is based on miscommunication in the parents' response to the infant's primary aggression at a very early stage of child development (as detailed further below), the former is a reaction to a loss of something good that has been positive in the child's experience up to a certain date and that has been withdrawn. The withdrawal of this good thing has extended over a period of time longer than that over which the child can keep

DOI: 10.4324/9781003466857-3

the memory of the positive experience alive (Winnicott et al. 2012/1984, p. 106). Stealing and destructiveness are emerging trends in antisocial tendency. From the deprived person's perspective, stealing involves the act of looking for something or someone. After not finding it/them, they look elsewhere in search of claiming what belongs to their natural right. Destructiveness, however, emerges from the desperate search for stability, for an environmental provision that could be able to re-establish the ego's needs whilst facilitating the emergence of the true self. Hence, the antisocial tendency can be perceived as inherent in normal emotional development, and above all as a sign that the child/young person has not yet given up hope of recovering what has been lost. According to Winnicott et al. (2012/1984), children or youths with anti-social tendencies underwent failures in their environment that have triggered difficulties in their maturational progress. Nevertheless, if one can provide new and stable environment provision, in which the child will be able to re-experiment his/her id impulses and/or aggressiveness in a frame of ego-relat-edness, then there is a chance that the tendency of being and becoming alive will be set in motion. 'In a frame of ego-relatedness, id-relationships occur and strengthen rather than disrupt the immature ego' (Winnicott 1958, p. 420). This ego-relatedness frame should be encouraged from the therapist's side by providing the child with ego support. However, the therapist should be able to endure repeated attacks.

> The analytic 'good object' is not someone better than the original object: it is someone who survives being treated as a 'bad object'. By surviving I mean neither collapsing under that experience nor retaliating because of it.
> (Casement 1991, pp. 269–270)

2 Aggression: A prism and its positive facet

Aggression itself is an iridescent conception. Depending on the point of view, different facets emerge, just like in a prism. For the concept of T-WAS, five facets were picked out: the violence facet, the social facet, the biological facet, the psychological facet and the positive facet.

Violence as a facet is adopted to draw attention to the difference between aggression as an experienced emotion and acting out of aggressive behaviour. It is true that aggression can be distinguished from violence. Nevertheless, it is still linked to violence, as it can be perceived as a component of it. Hacker has stressed that 'not all aggression is violence, but violence is always con-nected with aggression' (Hacker 1979, p. 13).

Gilligan (2001) emphasised that the purpose of violence is to enforce respect from others. According to him, shame is the arouser that triggers violence, and the extent to which a person feels shame depends on two vari-ables: the external one, which is based on the way other people treat you, and the internal one – the extent to which you are already self-conscious or ashamed of yourself. The external variable plays a central role, since it triggers a miscommunication between inner and external reality – a similar viewpoint to that of Winnicott and to Oaklander (1988, pp. 206–207). The more a person is shamed by others (from childhood by parents or peers) who ridicule or reject them, the more likely they are to feel shame. The less self-esteem one feels, the more one depends on the respect of others. The lack of a certain minimum level of respect from others or from one's self leads to a dead, uncaring and empty self within.

Like Gilligan, the neurobiologist Bauer (2011) emphasises the interpersonal level by writing: 'Aggression indicates that an individual experiencing pain or exclusion is unwilling and unable to accept social rejection inflicted upon him or her' (Bauer 2011, p. 63).

On top of this, the social facet strongly emphasises the negative role of aggression, which elicits social disapproval and is judged to be destructive and harmful in its consequences. Although social norms vary greatly depending on the cultural context, their authoritative feature is conformity pressure according to the motto: Control yourself!

The biological facet views aggression as an internal energy necessary for survival, which is released significantly by external stimuli. It is part of the human genetic make-up, which is also under the influence of hormonal fluctuations (Englander 2003; Krahé 2012; Perls et al. 1994).

Psychological approaches see aggression predominantly as a reaction to frustration, as an effect triggered by a negative stimulus. In epistemological psychoanalysis, it involves a destructive instinct. Aggression is also categorised as a conditioned behaviour, a result of social learning, which comes about through various reinforcing factors, through innumerable variables that influence the personal and social environment. In this respect, a number of authors, e.g., Bach and Goldberg (1976), Blom (2006), Casriel (1972), Winnicott et al. (2012/1984), Perls et al. (1994) and Mann (2020), regarded the interplay between social, biological and psychological aspects of aggression as critical to the understanding of its nature. Hence, they concluded on a more positive facet of it as described below.

For the positive facet, the energy of aggression is expressed on two levels: the individual level (through experiencing one's own anger) and the interpersonal level (through dealing with anger in conflict with others). The suppression of aggression energy on the individual level can constrain access to other feelings, impair awareness of one's own needs and restrict the experience of one's own anger, which in turn has an impact on the interpersonal level (Bittner 2018).

Perls et al. (1994) asserted that the way the word 'aggression' is used in gestalt includes 'everything that an organism does to initiate contact with its environment' (p. 70). Likewise, Mann (2020, pp. 285–286) emphasised that 'we need aggression to mobilise, move into action and make good contact'. Woods (1996, p. 83) stated that 'the capacity for violence has survival value'.

Casriel (1972), for example, suggested a clear emotional mapping of five elementary feelings: joy, love, pain, fear and anger. He assigns joy and love to positive feelings and fear and pain to negative ones. The fifth feeling, anger, is of central importance, similar to a switch. Accordingly, if anger is supressed, the feelings of pain and fear will come to the forefront and the supressed anger might eventually be expressed in the form of aggressive behaviour (i.e., escalation of conflict towards aggression/violence or somatisation, turning inwards). However, if one can clearly identify anger as a common feeling early on, and also express it in a controlled way, usually when it is triggered in conflict with others (by acknowledging it to the other person while seeking clarification through dialogue), one is more likely to be able to transform it into positive feelings, with joy and love coming to the fore.

> In our culture, almost everyone has some trouble giving and receiving anger. It is a constantly stifled feeling. Yet psychologically it is impossible to love someone without feeling angry at him quite frequently. If the anger is not shown, it has to be bottled up. And bottled-up anger leaks out as hostility, boredom, depression.
>
> (Casriel 1972, p. 76)

Bach and Goldberg (1976) have further deepened the understanding of how to deal constructively with aggressive energy. 'Aggressive energy, as we see it, can add a vital dimension to the process of living. That is, it can, when expressed constructively, intensify the depth and authenticity of personal and interpersonal relationships and experiences' (p. 114).

Together, Bach and Goldberg developed family therapy methods to address the suppressed energy of aggression from the individual level into an interpersonal setting. This led to the introduction of new, playful and body expression-oriented forms of conflict resolution between family members, such as the use of foam bats – batacas (see detailed practice guidance in chapter 7). In this context, they stress, for example, the educational value of parental resistance, which is essential for children to learn how to deal with their own aggressive energies. To do this constructively, parents should be aware of their own anger expression and be able to use it in a mastered way, and not 'take it out' on their children. Boundaries should be based on love, respect and self-control and should not be accompanied by doubts or feelings of guilt. Being aware of the reason for setting boundaries is essential (Castrechini-Franieck 2022; Woods 1993). Blom (2006) emphasised the need to set boundaries during Gestalt therapy so that the child can feel safe to express his or her feelings openly (more about Gestalt therapy settings can be found in chapter 2). 'Boundaries and limitations are necessary during the therapeutic process... This gives structure to the development of the therapeutic relationship, since growth cannot take place within a chaotic disorganized relationship' (p. 61), 'These boundaries are not aimed at punishing or restricting the child's emotional and physical security' (p. 64).

In line with Winnicott et al. (2012/1984, p. 99), one could summarise:

> the child whose home fails to give a feeling of security looks outside his home for the four walls; he still has hope, and he looks to grandparents, uncles, aunts, friends of family, school. He seeks an external stability without which he may go mad. Provided at the proper time, this stability might have grown into the child like the bones in his body, so that gradually in the course of the first months and years of his life he would have passed on to independence from dependence and a need to be managed. Often a child gets from the relations and school what he missed in his own actual home.

That is, antisocial acts/behaviours or delinquency are a result of a miscommunication in the early interaction between parents and child. Winnicott (2014) referred to a primary aggression – an original fusion of love and aggression – that is present at birth to assert itself in the world, the quality of which changes over the course of life. The role of the environment, which is initially family-based, is to nurture and help the child to experience this primary aggression in relationships, and this involves establishing boundaries and experiencing frustration as a result. In a healthy environment, primary aggression can be expressed, acted out and sublimated. If this is not the case, and the primary aggression is perceived as 'cruel, dangerous, hurtful' (preconcepts on the parents' part), then the child has to suppress it and cannot fully develop its 'self'. The resulting feeling of insecurity lays the emotional basis for antisocial acts/behaviours or delinquency.

For Winnicott et al. (2012/1984), the inner and outer worlds interact with each other and are in a constant dialogue of needs – in this sense, it seems similar to homeostasis as understood in Gestalt therapy (Blom 2006; Mann 2020; Perls et al. 1994). In Gestalt therapy, homeostasis means that the inner world is constantly negotiating which needs come to the fore (details in chapter 2).

Winnicott suggested that the treatment of the child at risk of antisocial tendency can be achieved by providing a nurturing environment ('neutral space') where the child can experiment, act out their primary aggressions and test their limits – the space that the child naturally and unconsciously seeks.

According to Woods (1996, p. 83), group work can contribute to the processing of violence if the therapist's own ability to tolerate and transform violent impulses is developed. The latter might be perceived as the attempt to find a container as referred to by Bion (1984a; 1984b), whereby Bion adds the process of 'maternal reverie' as described in chapter 2.

Wheeler (2006, p. 32) asserted: 'Social relations and their processes in complexly organised social groups – this is the ecological niche of human beings, and this is thus also the context in which human aggression is to be seen' (Wheeler, 2006, p. 32 – translation Bittner & Castrechini-Franieck).

Group work is therefore a good way to accompany relational processes within a protected setting. In this sense, it is a place of communal experience, particularly in dealing with anger.

Lucas (1988) took Winnicott's view that only from a position of shared reality can the individual clarify the boundary between inner and external reality, and she connected it to the principles of group analysis. She suggested that group psychotherapy based on group psychoanalytical principles for children can provide a new and stable environment (a 'holding' environment) in which the children may be triggered into a new cycle of maturational progress. However, adaptations should suit the age group as well as the institutional setting.

Castrechini-Franieck and Bittner (2022) took Winnicott's view of primary aggression and connected it with 'shared meaning communication'. As previously outlined, primary aggression is understood as an original fusion of love and aggression – an ambiguity per se. Hence, the achievement of 'shared meaning communication' should be related to the acknowledgment of the existence of primary aggression, which may succeed by consciously dealing with it in a neutral space in interaction with other group members (p. 162). Castrechini-Franieck and Bittner communicated, critically, the need for the adoption of an experiential approach that would allow the children to re-experiment the fusion of their feelings of love and aggression in a safe family-based environment whilst providing them with the chance of being and becoming alive – similar to an ego relatedness frame in the words of Winnicott (1958).

Whenever the authors refer to the term 'ego-relatedness' in this manuscript, it will always be in this sense.

James (1982) links the concept of transitional phenomena from Winnicott with the concept of matrix from Foulkes. In the same way that the child relates his/her inner world to the environment and people in it (external world), in group analysis, the individual relates to the group members via the matrix (or shared space).

3 Group matrix as referred to by Foulkes

Foulkes and Anthony (1990, p. 26) borrowed the insight from Gestalt therapy 'the whole is more elementary than the parts' to arrive at one of the basic concepts in the group work – the group should be perceived as a whole and not as a reunion of individual members. The network of all individual mental processes, the psychological medium in which they meet, communicate and interact, are referred to by Foulkes and Anthony as 'the matrix'. The term 'group matrix' describes the communication network among group members via interrelationships, interactions and modes of relatedness from distinct levels of relationships, for instance: intrapsychic, interpersonal and transpersonal. Foulkes (2018a; 2018b; Foulkes and Foulkes 1990) distinguished between a foundation group matrix, a personal group matrix and a dynamic one.

The foundation group matrix refers not only to the biological characteristics of the person but also includes cultural values and norms passed on by
family of origin, as well as by the social environment in which the person was
embedded (Foulkes 1992, pp. 131–132; see also Castrechini-Franieck 2017;
Franieck and Günter 2010) – some basic common ground.

Foulkes and Foulkes (1990, pp. 152–153) claimed that in the treatment
setting, all group members share certain general pre-conditioned ideas, such
as they should hold similar cultural backgrounds and should speak the same
language literally as well as metaphorically, otherwise the communication will
be inefficient. More simply, to build a group, all members should share a
similar foundation matrix.

The personal matrix is the sum of all an individual's relational experiences,
the representations of their own emotional experiences (Bion 1965) that are
passed on within group work.

The group dynamic matrix is perceived as the group's space, in which new
interrelationships, interactions, and modes of relatedness may trigger new and
corrective experiences, therefore impulses for inner change can emerge.
Foulkes and Anthony (1990) referred to this process as 'ego training in
action'. In this sense, the concept of a group dynamic matrix is somewhat
similar to the concept of a transitional space from Winnicott (1953), as
remarked by James (1982).

4 Some personal observations

Coping with antisocial tendencies (and/or behaviour) implies being faced with
aggression – antisocial tendency ties up essentially with aggression. Hence, to
develop a preventive group work with vulnerable children against the increase of
antisocial tendencies required being aware of the complex interplay between
aggression and love – the continual presence and acting out (expression) of the
primary aggression in-group. To put it another way, the group leaders should perceive aggression through the lens of a positive facet. At the same time, they should
maintain the ability to tolerate and transform violent impulses. For instance,
ambiguous feelings should be welcomed, jointly handled, mastered and promptly
integrated in-group via an accurate communication. By means of continuous
creative games, a secure ego-relationship structure within the group can be provided. In this manner, new experiences of self in relation to others can be undergone
in a playful transitional space (in line with Winnicott) or in a group matrix (in
accordance with Foulkes), and thereby resulting in a 'training of the ego in action'.

References

Bach, G.R., and Goldberg, H., 1976. *Creative Aggression*. London: Coventure.
Bauer, J., 2011. *Schmerzgrenze: Vom Ursprung alltäglicher und globaler Gewalt*. 3rd
    ed. München: Blessing.

Bion, W.R., 1965. *Transformations: Change from Learning to Growth*. London: William Heinemann Medical Books.

Bion, W.R., 1984a. *Attention & Interpretation*. London: Maresfield Reprints.

Bion, W.R., 1984b. *Learning from Experience*. London: Maresfield.

Bittner, N., 2018. *Junge männliche Gewalttäter: Aggressiv sein?! Erfahrungen zu Wutausdruck und Impulskontrolle*. Wald-Michelbach: Odenwald-Institut.

Blom, R., 2006. *The Handbook of Gestalt Play Therapy: Practical Guidelines for Child Therapists*. London: Jessica Kingsley Publishers.

Casement, P., 1991. *Learning from the Patient*. New York, London: Guilford Press.

Casriel, D., 1972. *A Scream Away from Happiness*. New York: Grosset & Dunlap.

Castrechini-Franieck, L., 2022. *Communication with Vulnerable Patients: A Novel Psychological Approach*. London: Routledge.

Castrechini-Franieck, L., and Bittner, N., 2022. T-WAS: Together We Are Strong. In L. Castrechini-Franieck (ed.), *Communication with Vulnerable Patients: A Novel Psychological Approach*. London: Routledge, 155–185.

Castrechini-Franieck, M.L., 2017. Wohin gehöre ich eigentlich? *JuKiP – Ihr Fachmagazin für Gesundheits- und Kinderkrankenpflege*, 6 (1), 36–39.

Englander, E.K., 2003. *Understanding Violence*. 2nd ed. Mahwah, NJ: Lawrence Erlbaum Associates.

Foulkes, S.H., 1992. *Gruppenanalytische Psychotherapie*. München: Pfeiffer.

Foulkes, S.H., 2018a. *Group-Analytic Psychotherapy: Method and Principles*. London: Routledge.

Foulkes, S.H., 2018b. *Therapeutic Group Analysis*. London: Routledge.

Foulkes, S.H., and Anthony, E.J., 1990. *Group Psychotherapy: The Psychoanalytic Approach*. 2nd ed. London: Routledge.

Foulkes, S.H., and Foulkes, E., 1990. *Selected Papers of S.H. Foulkes: Psychoanalysis and Group Analysis*. Edited and with a brief biography by E. Foulkes. London: Karnac Books.

Franieck, L., and Günter, M., 2010. *On Latency: Individual Development, Narcissistic Impulse Reminiscence and Cultural Ideal*. London: Routledge.

Gilligan, J., 2001. *Preventing Violence*. London: Thames & Hudson.

Hacker, F., 1979. *Aggression. Die Brutalisierung der modernen Welt*. 94th ed. Reinbek bei Hamburg: Rowohlt.

James, D.C., 1982. Transitional phenomena and the matrix in group psychotherapy. In M. Pines and L. Rafaelsen, ed., *The Individual and the Group*. New York: Plenum Press, 645–661.

Krahé, B., 2012. *The Social Psychology of Aggression*. 2nd ed. Hove: Psychology.

Lucas, T., 1988. Holding and holding-on: Using Winnicott's ideas in group psychotherapy with twelve- to thirteen-year-olds. *Group Analysis*, 21 (2), 135–149.

Mann, D., 2020. *Gestalt Therapy: 100 Key Points & Techniques*. 2nd ed. London: Routledge.

Oaklander, V., 1988. *Windows to Our Children: A Gestalt Therapy Approach to Children and Adolescents*. Highland, NY: Center for Gestalt Development.

Ogden, T.H., 2019. Ontological psychoanalysis or 'what do you want to be when you grow up?' *The Psychoanalytic Quarterly*, 88 (4), 661–684.

Perls, F.S., Hefferline, R., and Goodman, P., 1994. *Gestalt Therapy: Excitement and Growth in the Human Personality*. Highland, NY: Gestalt Journal Press.

Wheeler, G., 2006. Die Zukunft der Aggression: Eine gestalttherapeutische Meditation – Menschliche Natur, Theorie und Politik. In M.R. Staemmler, ed., *Aggression, Selbstbehauptung, Zivilcourage. Zwischen Destruktivität und engagierter Menschlichkeit.* Bergisch Gladbach: EHP Edition Humanistische Psychologie, 14–38.

Winnicott, D.W., 1953. Transitional objects and transitional phenomena: A study of the first not-me possession. *International Journal of Psycho-Analysis*, 34, 89–97.

Winnicott, D.W., 1958. The capacity to be alone. *International Journal of Psycho-Analysis*, 39, 416–420.

Winnicott, D.W., *et al.*, eds., 2012/1984. *Deprivation and Delinquency.* Abingdon: Routledge.

Winnicott, D.W., 2014. Aggression in relation to emotional development. In D.W. Winnicott, ed., *Collected Papers: Through Paediatrics to Psycho-Analysis.* London: Routledge, 204–217.

Woods, J., 1993. Limits and structure in child group psychotherapy. *Journal of Child Psychotherapy*, 19 (1), 63–78.

Woods, J., 1996. Handling violence in child group therapy. *Group Analysis*, 29 (1), 81–98.

Chapter 2

Relating Gestalt therapy to ontological psychoanalysis

This chapter brings together Gestalt therapy and ontological psychoanalysis and outlines their intersection point – the starting-point of the approach introduced in this book's manuscript, T-WAS (Together We Are Strong).

1 The child in Gestalt therapy

Gestalt therapy emphasises that all personal growth is regulated by a process called organismic self-regulation (or homeostasis). This is an ongoing process that supports the interplay between the demands of the individual and the outside world, and strives for balance as the outside world constantly challenges the individual. This process requires initiative and energy on the part of the individual to keep going, which in Gestalt therapy is referred to as 'aggressive (or survival) energy'. This not only regulates the expression of emotions, but also supports the self to remain in contact with itself while acting. For instance, when children are acting aggressively and fighting for control, often they experience a lack of this energy as they are acting beyond their limits. To put it another way, aggressive energy should not be mistaken for aggressive, hostile behaviour, as it is important for children to learn to express their spectrum of feelings. This is the starting point for the creative aggression approach mentioned in the previous chapter.

If the process of self-regulation is disturbed, inappropriate behaviours may arise and as a result, the ability to interact effectively with the environment may be impaired, leading not to a better life but rather to more difficulties (Perls et al. 1994). Take the case of a child who receives feedback from the environment that his or her personal way of creating balance is rejected; imbalance may be triggered. As a result, his or her aggressive energy will seek an alternative avenue to express itself, either turned inwards or outwards. Turned inwards, it resembles swallowing at a metabolic level, which then causes behaviours such as encapsulation – an excessive form of withdrawal. It may express itself, for example, in the form of numbing or 'dreaming away'. The aggressive energy may also increasingly go outwards, at the metabolic level, similar to vomiting, the expelling movement (Bittner 2021). Within such

DOI: 10.4324/9781003466857-4

cases, it expresses itself either in the form of striking behaviour by motor restlessness up to hyperactivity or antisocial plus violent behaviour.

> The way children express their emotions is related to their process and is often expressed in their behaviour rather than in their verbalisation.
>
> (Blom 2006, p. 123)

The assumption in Gestalt therapy is that children will manage their self-regulation by playing, which is the interface between inner and outer reality, so that competence in playing is also perceived as a life competence in itself (Oaklander 1981, p. 217). Training of perception via contact functions is regarded as an essential basis of emotional expression. Contact functions are understood as the abilities to see, hear, smell, taste, touch, move and form thoughts, ideas and opinions while learning to express and to define oneself through them (Oaklander 2001). Following the organismic self-regulation concept, the training of the contact functions is perceived to be a natural need and not supporting them is seen as a weakening of the self.

By means of facilitated play with an adult (therapist) who brings their experiences into play, aspects of the child's self – for example, being able / not being able, dealing with fantasies, power/curiosity, what belongs to me / what belongs to you, where do I belong, what am I allowed to do / what am I not allowed to do, etc. – can be consciously addressed with the aim of coming to terms with them. During this process, many aspects may be experienced in oppositional mode, as polarities. Approaching the middle from the poles and being able to cope with states of tension grow into one of the core aims of Gestalt therapy. Using creative, playful methods, it is possible to support the verbal and non-verbal expression of aggressive energy as well as emotional expression as a whole. This reinforces holistic self-regulation and therefore turns Gestalt therapy into a valuable approach for promoting resilience (Blom 2006; Hoosain 2009).

Being a facilitating therapist means being simply there, without imposing anything of one's own, but methodically inserting oneself into the child's rhythm with their full attention. In the encounter with the children, this dialogue attitude includes a positive view of the child's creative potential and the acceptance of the child without expectations. This attitude is also expressed in the therapist's interested and approachable manner, as well as in the therapist's feeling of responsibility for the protective setting. In summary, the purpose of Gestalt therapy is to integrate all dimensions of the child: to encourage the child's senses, body, emotions and mind to work in harmony, to promote the child's ability to self-regulate ('homeostasis') and to foster autonomy. 'The focus should be to guide the children towards awareness of polarities within themselves and in their lives, so that they may integrate them by making choices regarding handling them and taking responsibility for them' (Blom 2006, p. 41).

Children do spontaneously seek the group learning field by expressing and demanding their need for playing partners (Franck, 1997, pp. 16–17; Oaklander, 1981, p. 354), just as, incidentally, a major part of human life takes place in groups. In Gestalt therapy, (children's) groups are viewed as a social organism where the described learning processes of homeostasis, perception training and aggression processing take place among all group members. Therefore, a group represents a multifaceted field of learning. In this sense it is somewhat similar to the concepts of group matrix from Foulkes (2018a; 2018b; Foulkes and Foulkes 1990) and potential space from Winnicott (1953), as referred to in the previous chapter.

Unlike the epistemological psychoanalytical perspective, which focuses more on the transference processes within relationships, in Gestalt play therapy, these are not seen as paramount. Instead, it is about clarifying the role of the therapist to the child, in particular that the therapist does not perform the role of a parent (Oaklander 2001).

2 Communication by ontological psychoanalysis

The ontological-psychoanalytic perspective, for which, according to Ogden (2019), Winnicott and Bion are the main 'architects', emphasises experiential knowledge more than explanatory and reasoning knowledge, as is the case with the epistemic-psychoanalytic perspective, for which Freud and Klein are the main authors. Whereas the latter has the understanding of the unconscious inner world and its relation to the outer world as its object, the former reveals to the patient the experience of discovering a meaning for themselves and thereby finding themselves entirely. To illustrate, whilst Klein (1955) focused on the symbolic meaning of play, Winnicott (2005) emphasised the experience of being involved in play.

Stern et al.'s (1998) article 'Non-interpretive mechanisms in psychoanalytic therapy' marks a milestone in psychoanalysis, one that may also be considered as the starting point towards an ontological understanding of psychoanalysis. Based on research findings, the essence of therapeutic change is discussed in a new manner. In this article, the authors suggested two elements of change in analytic treatment: 1) interpretations, which re-arrange the intrapsychic landscape via insight (and are associated with the verbal realm, conscious) and declarative knowledge; and 2) 'moments of meeting', which bring about changes in relational quality via authentic interpersonal encounters, as well as experiences, and are linked to the relational domain. The latter are based on a sense of mutual understanding – referred to as 'shared implicit relationship'.

> 'Moments of meeting' are novel, personal, 'more' than transference interpretations, spontaneous, transcend but do not abrogate the professional relationship and are somewhat 'freed' from transference and

countertransference overtones. Stern views 'moments of meeting' as the nodal events of treatment.

(Williams 2011, p. 199)

Winnicott's concepts of 'holding' and 'transitional phenomena' can be related to the concept of 'moments of meeting'.

Holding, for Winnicott, is an ontological concept that he uses to explore the specific qualities of the experience of being alive at different developmental stages as well as the changing intrapsychic–interpersonal means by which the sense of continuity of being is sustained over time.

(Ogden 2004, p. 1350)

The first, bodily-emotional form of 'holding' is to ensure the basis of the infant's continuing being, characterised by 'primary maternal preoccupation' – the mother 'feels herself taking the place of the infant' (Winnicott 2014, p. 304), which is the essence of the process of 'mutuality'.

'Mutuality' is described as the mother's ability to identify with her baby, whereas the baby feels himself to be understood – a product of unconscious communication and feelings shaped between the infant and his mother. Thus, the experience of mutuality can be perceived as an interdependent two-way process. On the one hand, there is the mother and her identification with her infant, and on the other hand, there is the infant with his inner potential to grow (an achievement for the baby).

(Castrechini-Franieck 2022, p. 18)

However, inevitable circumstances will arise that will also result in experiences of maternal failure. Such experiences will be perceived by the infant as a threat to its personal existence, paradoxically, however, they will also enable the infant to exist, to experience, to master instincts and to build a personal self. The latter can be understood as the internalisation of the primary function of the mother's initial circumferential physical-psychological 'holding'. It also involves making the effects of time on the infant bearable (transforming the infant's timelessness) and thus establishing the illusion of a world in which time is measured. As the infant grows, the function of 'holding' changes from that of protecting the infant's body to one of maintaining/supporting more objective forms of being alive throughout time. Part of these maintenance forms includes the provision of a 'place' (a psychological state), a 'neutral/ potential space', where the infant may find itself. Providing this psychological space depends on the ability of the other person to tolerate the 'unknown feeling' associated with 'coming together in one place' (Winnicott 2014), or in accordance with Stern et al. (1998), on the quality of the relationship in 'moments of meeting'.

According to Ogden (2004) Winnicott's most important contribution to an ontological understanding of psychoanalysis consists of the concepts of 'transitional objects' and 'transitional phenomena'. From the clinical point of view, the transitional object can be conceptualised essentially as the object that not only permeates the communication between the inner and outer worlds, but also forms the transition between fantasy and reality (by embracing the difference and similarity between the two), while also enabling symbolism (Castrechini-Franieck 2022). Winnicott (1953) viewed the transitional phenomenon experience as the creation of an 'illusory experience' – a third area of experience between fantasy and reality; as a facet of the internalisation process of maternal 'holding', an emotional situation in time.

Bion's idea of 'container-contained' is often used interchangeably with Winnicott's idea of 'holding', however both ideas are based on different kinds of analytical thinking (Crepaldi 2018; Ogden 2004). Whereas Winnicott's idea of 'holding' primarily emphasises the mother–infant interaction on the sensory-mediated level (processes that belong to the 'external reality'), Bion's idea about the interdependent process of 'container-contained interaction' places attention on the inner psychological developing skills of dreaming, digesting and thinking (Bion 1984a; 1984b). In other words, on the dynamic interplay between the thoughts and feelings arising from the emotional experience lived or contained process. In the beginning, the primitive, still purely physical-emotional experiences that humans undergo have to be Contained, i.e., held, to be experienced meaningfully and gradually give rise to thoughts as a third element. Parents, on their part, process the impressions they get from their infant, provide themselves as containers and return their impressions to their child in a transformed format. As already mentioned, the interaction between container and child involves three processes of developing thought: 1) unconscious dreaming, 2) preconscious reverie, and 3) conscious reflection, which drives the process of the container. Put more simply: 1) the ability to dream, to be empathetic to the unconscious, 2) the ability to take all these dreams and digest them – the ' maternal reverie' – and 3) bringing them to a conscious reflection process in order to develop thoughts further. 'Maternal reverie' is therefore central to this process, and it is described in more detail as the ability to sense (and understand) what is going on inside the infant (client/group/counterpart). It is 'the mother's capacity to contain her child's primitive communication whilst transforming sense information or misrepresented/disorganized experiences (beta elements) into creative thinking (alpha elements), which will provide the mind with a thinking apparatus' (Castrechini-Franieck, 2022, p. 17).

From Bion's point of view, psychoanalysis should not focus on the symbolic meaning of dreams and their interpretation, but on the mutual resonance of the dreams presented by the client, which arises from the encounter between analyst and client. He conceived dream work as a fundamental model of the functioning of the human psyche, which is in no way bound only to sleep, but exhibits multiple emotional manifestations. The analyst's role is thus to deal with the dynamic between beta and alpha elements triggered by the encounter between the two – analyst and client – a process described by Cassorla (2018) as 'analyst daydreaming'.

It is worth underlining that Bion worked with groups as a social scientist under the influence of John Rickman at a time when he was not yet a qualified psychoanalyst. It is true that he developed some concepts on group dynamics from his work with groups, which have contributed to an understanding about organisational development processes (Hinshelwood 2007). Nonetheless, the authors have intentionally decided to only refer to his ideas of 'container' and 'maternal reverie' owing to the features of the group as described above.

Reviewing, the epistemological psychoanalysis involves primarily the search for understanding unconscious meaning content. The goal of ontological psychoanalysis, in turn, is to enable patients to discover meaning content creatively and become fully alive through this process (Ogden 2019, p. 665).

3 Some personal observations

The intersection point between ontological psychoanalysis and Gestalt therapy is located in the therapist's role on two levels – the first level as being someone who accepts the child as he/she is, without holding expectations, and the second level as being a facilitator, or a provider of a space (a neutral/potential one) within the relationship, in which the child is enabled to experiment, to act out his/her blurred/ambiguous feelings, although limits may be tested and responsibilities may be taken. In fact, both theoretical frameworks share the same goal, which is to guide the child towards integration, thereby finding him/herself entirely. Another intersection point concerns their understanding of aggression as a positive facet. However, they handle the communication with the child differently by adopting particular approaches. Whilst Gestalt therapy lays emphasis on the training of the contact functions, promoting catharsis while denying transference and counter-transference issues, the ontological psychoanalysis lays stress on the 'moment of meeting', 'holding', 'mutuality', 'transitional object', 'transitional space', 'maternal reverie' and 'container-contained' – psychological/emotional states experienced in the relationship are the focus, including all possibilities of 'analyst daydreaming' (Cassorla 2018). Another differential is related to the therapy session structure. In Gestalt therapy, with the aim of attaining homeostasis, the therapist may encourage the patient to experiment with (mostly) cathartic exercises to release negative feelings whilst coming into contact with them – the same for adults and children. In psychoanalysis the 'free-association' principle is imperative. The therapist therefore remains neutral, as well as attentive to the patients' discourse, whilst abstaining from any kind of interference on the free association process. In the case of children, the child holds the free will to decide what to play; there is no encouragement on the part of the therapist to start a play. The approach to group work with vulnerable children outlined in this book, Together We Are Strong or T-WAS, emerges from the intersection of Gestalt therapy and ontological psycho-analysis and deals with group communications by looking at both of these methods.

References

Bion, W.R., 1984a. *Learning from experience*. London: Maresfield.

Bion, W.R., 1984b. *Second Thoughts: Selected Papers on Psychoanalysis*. London: Routledge.

Bittner, N., 2021. *Kontakt, Spiel, Aggression und Gruppe. Aspekte des Werdens durch Gestalt*. Unpublished final dissertation, Tübingen.

Blom, R., 2006. *The Handbook of Gestalt Play Therapy: Practical Guidelines for Child Therapists*. London: Jessica Kingsley Publishers.

Cassorla, R.M.S., 2018. *The Psychoanalyst, the Theatre of Dreams and the Clinic of Enactment*. Abingdon, New York, NY: Routledge.

Castrechini-Franieck, L., 2022. *Communication with Vulnerable Patients: A Novel Psychological Approach*. London: Routledge.

Crepaldi, G., 2018. *Containing*. Giessen: Psychosozial-Verlag.

Foulkes, S.H., 2018a. *Group-Analytic Psychotherapy: Method and Principles*. London: Routledge.

Foulkes, S.H., 2018b. *Therapeutic Group Analysis*. London: Routledge.

Foulkes, S.H., and Foulkes, E., 1990. *Selected Papers of S.H. Foulkes: Psychoanalysis and Group Analysis*. Edited and with a brief biography by E. Foulkes. London: Karnac Books.

Franck, J., 1997. *Gestalt-Gruppentherapie mit Kindern*. 1st ed. Freiamt: Arbor-Verl.

Hinshelwood, R.D., 2007. Bion and Foulkes: The group-as-a-whole. *Group Analysis*, 40 (3), 344–356.

Hoosain, S., 2009. *Resilience in Refugee Children: A Gestalt Play Therapy Approach*. Master's degree, University of South Africa.

Klein, M., 1955. The psychoanalytic play technique. *American Journal of Orthopsychiatry*, 25 (2), 223–237.

Oaklander, V., 1981. *Gestalttherapie mit Kindern und Jugendlichen*. Stuttgart: Klett-Cotta.

Oaklander, V., 2001. Gestalt play therapy. *International Journal of Play Therapy*, 10, 45–55.

Ogden, T.H., 2004. On holding and containing, being and dreaming. *The International Journal of Psychoanalysis*, 85 (6), 1349–1364.

Ogden, T.H., 2019. Ontological psychoanalysis or 'what do you want to be when you grow up?' *The Psychoanalytic Quarterly*, 88 (4), 661–684.

Perls, F.S., Hefferline, R., and Goodman, P., 1994. *Gestalt Therapy: Excitement and Growth in the Human Personality*. Highland, NY: Gestalt Journal Press.

Stern, D.N., *et al.*, 1998. Non-interpretive mechanisms in psychoanalytic therapy: The 'something more' than interpretation. *The International Journal of Psychoanalysis*, 79 (5), 903–921.

Williams, A., 2011. *Working with Street Children: An Approach Explored.* Lyme Regis: Russell House.
Winnicott, D.W., 1953. Transitional objects and transitional phenomena: A study of the first not-me possession. *International Journal of Psycho-Analysis,* 34, 89–97.
Winnicott, D.W., 2005. *Playing and reality.* London: Routledge.
Winnicott, D.W., 2014. Primary maternal preoccupation. In D.W. Winnicott, ed., *Collected Papers: Through Paediatrics to Psycho-Analysis.* London: Routledge, 300–305.

Chapter 3

Running a group in partnership
What does this mean?

This chapter highlights several different theoretical views on group leadership for children, which includes the type, size and structure of the group, and the group leader's role, whether single or in two leaderships. If the group is led by two people, attention is also given to the question of the difference between co-leadership and pair leadership in group work with children and their pros and cons. It lays the groundwork for the conceptualisation of the novel concept of 'eclectic group conductors' – one of the key pillars of T-WAS (Castrechini-Franieck and Bittner, 2022) – to be introduced in chapter 5.

1 Models of children's group work and the role of the group leader

The classical children's group work in Gestalt therapy, initiated by Oaklander (2001), used dream work and the empty chair technique. It presented itself as open to methods and also integrates, for example, the sandbox technique, as well as experiential approaches to promote self-support and expressiveness. Oaklander was also the one who worked on the principle of model learning, with a single child in front of the group, which can usually only be considered in very small groups of up to six children.

Wirth (2012a) emphasises that group work with children happens at a basal level, where non-verbal, primarily physical impulses of movement and expressiveness indicate ongoing development. The group represents the social field in which these child-typical movements can unfold. In this context, individual and social field forces may be perceived as polarities and dealing with them may be understood as a developmental task of the group work. These immediate expressions of the child also shape an orientation towards being in the present in group work. The child's existence is encouraged by what is continually happening and is being represented in the 'here and now'. As Franck (1997, p. 21) emphasised: 'the child experiences these figures and their actions with his or her full perception in the present'.

DOI: 10.4324/9781003466857-5

Running a group in partnership: What does this mean? 25

Besides an active, interested attitude, the group leader provides a safe setting and introduces developmental offers by means of materials while taking up the children's impulses to design the programme. The group leader encourages experiments and responds flexibly to the participants' needs so that the children's own resources can be applied. Thereby, the group leader shows themselves with their strengths and weaknesses so that relationships can be improved and a mutual understanding can be achieved within the group. For the group leadership, cultivating mindfulness, sociability and experimentation skills are key competences. In case of destructive expressions of aggressive energy, Franck (1997) recommended a basic reaction on the non-verbal communication level, such as the short-term use of a loud voice without speech content or even physical contact, in order to trigger a pause. By slowing down the process, the emotional perception of what is happening can generally be made available again (Franck 1997, pp. 68–69). Gestalt therapy group leaders in children's groups are flexible in moving back and forth between linguistic and non-linguistic levels of communication.

For a long time, psychodynamic group work with children has been shaped by the epistemic-psychoanalytic perspective (Slavson 1950; Slavson and Schiffer 1975) in addition to experiences with clinical target groups. Recently, however, several authors such as Lehle (2018); Brandes (2009); Lucas (1988); Woods (1996); Westman (1996); Moll (1997); and Ballhausen-Scharf et al. (2021) have focused on ontological-psychoanalytic thinking in group work.

Slavson (1950), who is considered the founder of psychodynamic child group psychotherapy (Heinemann and Horst 2009), emphasised the transferability of psychoanalytic concepts to group work with children. In his view, children can learn how to improve their behaviour especially in a peer group. He considered games in the group as the core means of therapy for facilitating the acting out of inner conflicts (via the catharsis process) while enabling them to further empathise with other group members (assisted by the sublimation process). In this way, he believed that a sense of belonging may be set up and the feeling of identity strengthened, thereby enabling the development of ego-strength and social competence. The groups he worked with were small and homogeneous (in terms of age, gender and symptomatology), with a maximum of eight participants. His approach deliberately set himself apart from educating adults by showing a self-direction in which the desired group norms appear, hence an educative effect after all. He also emphasised that each group member projects his or her unconscious image of an adult (parental idealisation) onto the therapist, in the sense of a transference concept (Slavson and Schiffer 1975, p. 132). Therefore, the role of the therapist or group leader should remain as neutral as possible, based on the principles of unconditional acceptance of the child and non-interference.

It was Anthony (Foulkes and Anthony 1990) who worked with smaller groups of children than Slavson (five to six participants), yet the participants had a wider range in terms of age, gender, temperament and diagnoses.

Potential disruptions triggered by the greater diversity were regarded as giving rise to issues in the group, whilst also developing the participants' coping skills, thus being perceived as having a positive effect. His focus was more on the group and its needs rather than on the therapist and matching the group to the therapist's skills. In particular, Anthony emphasised the fact that at the communication level, two elements should be seriously well thought out by the therapist:

1   Their ability for 'two-way communication' with the children – put more simply, the basic dialogical attitude in Gestalt therapy, the ability to engage as much as possible with a child as an equal and show interest in all expressive forms of the child, plus the ability to play with the child.
2   An emphasis on the importance of translating activity into language rather than interpreting it relates strongly to Bion's understanding of the primacy of relational affectivity as the origin of thinking rather than developing logical reasoning (Crepaldi 2018).

However, he drew attention to the fact that this active communication might increase the risk of the group leader being under the influence of counter-transference issues, as both positive and negative feelings towards the group members may naturally arise during the process of communication.

Foulkes (2018b, pp. 54–65); Foulkes and Foulkes 1990, pp. 285–296), in particular, regarded the leader as both a participant in the group and simultaneously as a 'conductor' (a role similar to a musical conductor who interprets the music, but does not compose it). The conductor sets the pace like a maestro while carefully playing along, depending on the situation. He lets the group lead; he intervenes with restraint and is aware of his impact on the group. As a member of the group, his personality is meaningful in the group, yet he uses it with restraint. Whenever the term 'group conductor' or 'conductor' is referred to in this manuscript, it will always be in this sense raised by Foulkes. In the German version of this book, the term 'group conductor' was replaced with '*Gruppe Leitung*'.

More authors have recently considered the ontological-psychoanalytic understanding as a means of improving communication in group work with children.

Brandes (2009) referred to a 'potential space' in the group, a transitional space (Winnicott 1995), where group members may bring in life-historically significant scenes and creatively process them.

As a Winnicott student, Hofmann (2010) transferred her child analytic experiences to the group analytic context. She emphasised the importance of emotional containment by the group leader (in the sense of 'holding') and of scenic play (in the form of group activities) for developing group cohesion and mentalisation processes.

Lehle (2018) and Ballhausen-Scharf et al. (2021) understood the group analytic process as a circular game that promotes the development of the individual as well as the group as a whole. The group leader's main task is to promote and ensure a potential transitional space for the group members in which they can come into contact with their inner and outer worlds (Winnicott 1953; Winnicott et al. 2012/1984). The task of the group leader is also, among other things, to assist in overcoming antisocial tendencies in the group by restoring a safe space within the group and its containment function. Through the addition of a verbal dimension to the destructive expressions, the ego function of the members is supported and therefore can be accessed both in the group process and by individual group members. Promoting and containing this circular interplay can be perceived as 'maternal reverie' (Bion 1984b).

Moll (1997) had raised the question of the effectiveness of children's group work when, in line with Stern (1998/1985; 2000/1995), her focus was on changes in relational representations. She noted that these are not triggered by verbalisation but rather more directly by the interactions within the relational group setting, particularly by processing feelings, or, in Gestalt terms, by promoting the formation of the contact functions. She viewed establishing 'moments of meeting' (Stern et al. 1998), as described in chapter 2, as an essential means for expanding the child's experiential and behavioural potential. She perceived the role and function of therapists as akin to Lehle (2018) and Ballhausen-Scharf et al. (2021).

Woods (1996) and Lucas (1988) worked in the group context specifically with vulnerable children with antisocial tendencies. Similar to the aforementioned authors, in the ontological-psychoanalytic approach, they found answers to their question as to how communication within the group can be managed (and properly comprehended).

Woods referred to Winnicott et al. (2012/1984) to explain the roots of aggression, its expression and its potential counteracting impact on the group leader. To give a meaningful framework to the level of aggression representation, Woods also referred to Bion's beta and alpha element dynamics (Bion 1984a).

Lucas underlined the parallel between the concepts of the 'matrix' (Foulkes 2018a; Foulkes 2018b; Foulkes and Foulkes 1990) and transitional phenomena (Winnicott 1953). She argued that children communicate with the environment and people through a 'shared space' while structuring their own internal object world. Therefore, therapy with vulnerable children with antisocial tendencies needs to be much more concrete and focused on here-and-now – quite similar thinking to that of Franck (1997) and Wirth (2012a, 2012b) in Gestalt therapy. She also suggested the introduction of games in the group in order to 'create space' in which the unconscious is triggered, allowing the expression of aggression while encouraging associative thinking. In this way, group members may experience phases of regression with which they struggle and which inhibit their growth. The essential quality of the therapist, for Lucas, is the ability to 'hold' (Winnicott 1960).

2 Co-leaders and pair-conductors ('Paarleitung') in children's group work

Cividini-Strani and Klain (1984) presented a detailed analysis of the pros and cons of co-leadership. However, they did not consider the gender aspect. They explored possible differences in experience levels between pairs of leaders (experienced-experienced, inexperienced-experienced, inexperienced-inexperienced) and went on to describe how these differences in experience levels might affect group leadership, together with possible strategies for avoiding such effects.

Foulkes (2018a, pp. 105–106) emphasised that a 'co-conductor' in the group – if there is one – should work well with the conductor and take on the role of an 'assistant', a pure 'observer', without disturbing or arousing suspicion through his or her presence in the group. Trautmann-Voigt and Voigt (2019) und Haar and Wenzel (2019) shared Foulke's perspective, although the former considered heterogeneity in leadership as a positive effect that makes the group more multifaceted and lively. For example, group members could explore playful attachments both with two different therapist personalities and in a triad (three-way relationship).

Nowadays, Gestalt therapists work with a co-leader in the adult group, in a similar role to that described by Foulkes. Oaklander (1981, p. 354) enjoyed working with another therapist, but there is no mention of how the shared workload was organised. In contrast, Franck (1997) preferred a mixed-gender pair of leaders in the children's group. His texts employ the pronoun 'we' indicating that the two would be a single unit. However, if a child is disruptive during the early stages of the group, he suggests that one of the leaders pay more attention to that child so that the child can join the group (Franck 1997, p. 69). This is what Rahm and Kirsch (1997) recommended for a group of children, and they had in mind only four to six children taking part in the group. In their opinion, a group leadership team should be considered. The leadership team should consist of two gender-diverse and experienced co-therapists (the main group leaders) and two trainees or educators. The latter are given a role where they can respond more to individual children during disruptions. A group leadership team has the advantage of ensuring the continuity of the group, even if one of the leaders is unavailable.

From a theoretical point of view, Slavson (1950, pp. 111–112) has a negative view of mixed gender leadership in children's groups. In his view, mixed gender leadership can not only lead to transference disorders; it can also confuse the children's reactions to the caregivers in the group. In practice, however, he made it clear that there is still a need to clarify the potential benefits of mixed-sex leadership as a means of reproducing the family environment.

Anthony (Foulkes and Anthony 1990, pp. 186, 230), on his part, emphasised that using therapists of different genders in leading children's groups can broaden the spectrum of treatment and is therefore an important component of the therapeutic work.

For Moll (1997), a mixed-gender pair of conductors was favourable, as the intention of group therapy is basically to address the children's needs in daily situations. A family-like relationship context in the group could support changes in relationship representations.

In group analysis with children and adolescents in German-speaking countries, the term 'Paarleitung' is currently preferred to emphasise the equality of the relationship between the leaders. The Anglo-American term 'co-leadership' does not take this aspect of the non-hierarchical relationship into account. The term 'Paarleitung' is linked to an extension of the children's developmental space, as it allows them to re-enact family experiences and to experience a three-person relationship (Ballhausen-Scharf et al. 2021; Hofmann 2010; Moll 1997; Trautmann-Voigt and Voigt 2019). From an ontological-psychoanalytic perspective, the emphasis is more on the common opportunity to offer new, positive attachment experiences rather than the re-enactment of them (Ogden 2019; Stern 2000/1995). Ballhausen-Scharf et al. (2021) pointed out that the nature of the relationship of the couple in the lead should not be hidden from the group. However, at the beginning of group processes, they recommended that disagreements between the 'couple leaders', especially about an appropriate course of action, should not be openly discussed in front of group members. Rather, the group should first have a sufficient degree of cohesion before such communication would be helpful for the group process. Then it could release constructive potential.

Westman (1996) worked with a co-therapy understanding and the concept of re-parenting with vulnerable children, and highlighted the significance and importance of communication between the therapists before, during and after the group work. She thought that this has a major impact on the group dynamics. Co-therapy has positive therapeutic potential if the tensions in co-leadership and with the children are carefully negotiated. The risk of over-idealising co-leadership and the likelihood of dependency and scapegoating is another point to consider.

3 Some personal observations

Overall, the authors share a common perspective on the role of the group leader in a group of children: a neutral person with the skills to promote a secure environment for children, in which the children may feel free to express themselves. Different perspectives are related to the group features as well as to the pair of group leaders. For the former, the groups can vary with regard to number of participants, similar or different diagnoses and the age range of the children. In general, small groups (no more than eight participants) are recommended. In terms of diagnosis and age range, it is clear that the greater the variation in these criteria, the more vulnerable the group is to disruption. The handling of this potential disruption will depend on the ability of the group leader to deal with conflicts and with what is unknown in the group.

The critical point in leading a group as a pair concerns the way in which leadership can be shared without creating personal competition between the leaders. Many conscious and unconscious variables may affect the partnership, apart from the qualities and skills of each leader in dealing with personal differences. Therefore, some authors considered it more appropriate to combine leadership with separate roles: a person in charge of the group and another in the position of observer or outsider. However, other authors have considered shared pair leadership as being very beneficial for group development. They have also stressed the influential variables that might be involved in the work of the pair and how they can be managed. However, there is still a lack of literature on the reporting of specific practical details experienced by group leaders when co-leading a group. This issue will be addressed by the authors in later chapters.

References

Ballhausen-Scharf, B., *et al.*, 2021. *Gruppenanalyse mit Kindern und Jugendlichen. Ein Leitfaden zur Kompetenzentwicklung.* Goettingen: Vandenhoeck & Ruprecht.

Bion, W.R., 1984a. *Attention & Interpretation.* London: Maresfield Reprints.

Bion, W.R., 1984b. *Learning from Experience.* London: Maresfield.

Brandes, H., 2009. Die Kindergruppe als Übergangsraum. *Gruppenprozesse unter Kider und Jugendlichen*, 32 (115), 49–60. www.psychosozial-verlag.de/26146.

Castrechini-Franieck, L., and Bittner, N., 2022. T-WAS: Together We Are Strong. In L. Castrechini-Franieck (ed.), *Communication with Vulnerable Patients: A Novel Psychological Approach.* London: Routledge, 155–185.

Cividini-Strani, E., and Klain, E., 1984. Advantages and disadvantages of co-therapy. *Group Analysis*, 17 (2), 156–159.

Crepaldi, G., 2018. *Containing.* Giessen: Psychosozial-Verlag.

Foulkes, S.H., 2018a. *Group-Analytic Psychotherapy: Method and Principles.* London: Routledge.

Foulkes, S.H., 2018b. *Therapeutic Group Analysis.* London: Routledge.

Foulkes, S.H., and Anthony, E.J., 1990. *Group Psychotherapy: The Psychoanalytic Approach.* 2nd ed. London: Routledge.

Foulkes, S.H., and Foulkes, E., 1990. *Selected Papers of S.H. Foulkes: Psychoanalysis and Group Analysis.* Edited and with a brief biography by E. Foulkes. London: Karnac Books.

Franck, J., 1997. *Gestalt-Gruppentherapie mit Kindern.* 1st ed. Freiamt: Arbor-Verl.

Haar, R., and Wenzel, H., 2019. *Psychodynamische Gruppentherapie mit Kindern.* 1st ed. Stuttgart: Kohlhammer.

Heinemann, C., and Horst, T.v.d., 2009. *Gruppenpsychotherapie mit Kindern. Ein Praxisbuch.* 1st ed. Stuttgart: Kohlhammer.

Hofmann, E., 2010. Gruppenanalytische Arbeit mit Kindern: Eine Gruppe wird 'geboren'. Stufen im Prozess zu einer ambulanten Kindergruppe. *Gruppenanalyse*, 20 (1), 53–81.

Lehle, H.G., 2018. 'Egotraining in Aktion'. Das Spiel in der psychoanalytischen Kindergruppentherapie. In B. Traxl, ed. *Psychodynamik im Spiel. Psychoanalytische*

Überlegungen und klinische Erfahrungen zur Bedeutung des Spiels. Frankfurt AM: Brandes & Apsel, 133–158.

Lucas, T., 1988. Holding and holding-on: Using Winnicott's ideas in group psychotherapy with twelve- to thirteen-year-olds. *Group Analysis*, 21 (2), 135–149.

Moll, M., 1997. Thesen zur gruppenanalytischen Arbeit mit Kindern. *Arbeitshefte Gruppenanalyse*, 12, 22–31.

Oaklander, V., 1981. *Gestalttherapie mit Kindern und Jugendlichen.* Stuttgart: Klett-Cotta.

Oaklander, V., 2001. Gestalt play therapy. *International Journal of Play Therapy*, 10, 45–55.

Ogden, T.H., 2019. Ontological psychoanalysis or 'what do you want to be when you grow up?' *The Psychoanalytic Quarterly*, 88 (4), 661–684.

Rahm, D., and Kirsch, C., 1997. *Integrative Gruppentherapie mit Kindern.* Göttingen: Vandenhoeck & Ruprecht.

Slavson, S.R., 1950. *Analytic Group Psychotherapy: With Children Adolescents and Adults.* New York: Columbia University Press.

Slavson, S.R., and Schiffer, M., 1975. *Group Psychotherapies for Children: A Textbook.* New York: International Universities Press.

Stern, D.N., 1998/1985. *The Interpersonal World of the Infant: A View from Psychoanalysis and Developmental Psychology.* London: Karnac Books.

Stern, D.N., 2000/1995. *The Motherhood Constellation: A Unified View of Parent-Infant Psychotherapy.* New York: Basic Books.

Stern, D.N., et al., 1998. Non-interpretive mechanisms in psychoanalytic therapy. The 'something more' than interpretation. *The International Journal of Psychoanalysis*, 79 (5), 903–921.

Trautmann-Voigt, S., and Voigt, B., eds., 2019. *Mut zur Gruppentherapie! Das Praxisbuch für gruppenaffine Psychotherapeuten: Leitfäden Interventionstipps Antragsbeispiele nach der neuen PT-Richtlinie.* Stuttgart: Schattauer.

Westman, A., 1996. Cotherapy and 're-parenting' in a group for disturbed children. *Group Analysis*, 29 (1), 55–68.

Winnicott, D.W., 1953. Transitional objects and transitional phenomena: A study of the first not-me possession. *International Journal of Psycho-Analysis*, 34, 89–97.

Winnicott, D.W., 1960. The theory of the parent-child relationship. *International Journal of Psycho-Analysis*, 41, 585–595.

Winnicott, D.W., 1995. *Vom Spiel zur Kreativität.* 8th ed. Stuttgart: Klett-Cotta.

Winnicott, D.W., et al., eds., 2012/1984. *Deprivation and Delinquency.* Abingdon: Routledge.

Wirth, W., 2012a. Entwicklungsbewegungen der Gestalttherapie. In H. Anger, ed., *Gestalttherapie mit Kindern und Jugendlichen.* Bergisch Gladbach: EHP, 15–48.

Wirth, W., 2012b. Gestalttherapie mit traumatisierten Kindern und Jugendlichen. In H. Anger, ed., *Gestalttherapie mit Kindern und Jugendlichen.* Bergisch Gladbach: EHP, 281–316.

Woods, J., 1996. Handling violence in child group therapy. *Group Analysis*, 29 (1), 81–98.

Part 2

Together We Are Strong (T-WAS)

Chapter 4

The challenges behind the scenes

Working in the psychosocial field necessarily entails being able to actively shape and (above all) maintain contact with the 'Other' person; it requires resources that go far beyond the study of books. Maintaining a balance between empathic contact with the 'Other' person and contact with one's own autonomy (e.g., accessing one's own free will) challenges the dimension of self-regulation (Mann 2020; Perls et al. 1994). It involves one's ability to allow oneself to undergo an emotional state in the interaction with the 'Other' without having the fear of losing oneself, nor of falling into rigid contact avoidance (Blankertz and Doubrawa 2017; Casement 1991), whilst keeping one's own balance on top of one's professionalism. Mastering this skill necessarily points toward being deeply aware of one's own personal history (one's own foundation matrix) before engaging in group work with vulnerable children. For the development of T-WAS, the awareness of the sui generis authors' biographies was crucial and, at the same time, the first challenge they met. Below, to illustrate this, a brief biography of the authors will be supplied to the reader. Moreover, the 'we'-form, and also the authors' first names 'Leticia' and 'Niko', will be preferably adopted in this book from now on.

I The foundation matrix of group conductors – the signatures are sui generis

I.I Leticia's foundation matrix – a short biography

Leticia grew up in Brazil, in a traditional middle-class family with Italian-Hispanic roots, at a time in which physical punishment was quite normal. She was the only girl among three brothers. She was brought up in the traditional role of housewife and mother. According to her representation of her emotional experiences (Bion 1965), her mother's entire attention was focused on the boys, and her own place in this family constellation remained unclear to her. To overcome this, Leticia invested all her energy in developing her cognitive abilities, achieving school results that were exemplary; after all, she wanted to find a place in the world where she could embody something

DOI: 10.4324/9781003466857-7

'worthwhile'. Her hobby during adolescence was to spend time solving mathematical equations – working with mathematical symbols and their meanings and arriving at a solution to or a representation of a problem was a challenge she really enjoyed. Perhaps on an unconscious emotional level, she was simply trying to find meaning where there was none – a kind of 'reverie function' as asserted by Bion (1984). In the abstract world of mathematics, Leticia found her recognition and became encapsulated in it. Her parents' relationship was constantly marked by conflict; the couple as a unit never existed in her view. The parental relationship finally broke down as a result of domestic violence once the children reached puberty – a difficult time for all family members. As a result, Leticia decided to do her analysis training as soon as she started her undergraduate studies in psychology. The feeling of being an 'outsider' in her own family was the central theme of it. This in turn awakened the desire in her to work with 'outsiders' herself. She therefore started working as a clinical psychologist at a psychiatric hospital and later trained as a psychodynamic psychotherapist, working in her own practice in Brazil. When she started her own family with a German-Brazilian man, she moved to Germany due to her husband's work. Her twin sons were already eight years old at the time and the change of culture and language was a daunting and challenging experience for everyone. Being an 'outsider' became a reality. Her children often experienced rejection from their peers at school and Leticia could not understand why children at this age could not just play together. Did the understanding and meaning of family, as well as the feeling of belonging to a group, have different values in Germany? In search of an answer to this question, Leticia began her academic career. Since then, Leticia has carried out studies into cultural issues and on vulnerable children. Her studies have been funded by the International Psychoanalytical Association (IPA) and have led to several publications: Franieck and Günter (2010); Castrechini-Franieck et al. (2014); Castrechini-Franieck (2017); Castrechini-Franieck and Page (2017). Her current clinical practice is focused on the social field, working with highly vulnerable populations, such as forensic patients with personality disorders, traumatised refugees and vulnerable children/youths. In her clinical work, she has an ontological-psychoanalytic background (Castrechini-Franieck 2022).

1.2 Niko's foundation matrix – a short biography

Niko initially grew up in two foster families in Germany before he was adopted at the age of seven. This was an incognito adoption, in which no knowledge of the family of origin was passed on to the adoptive family. These early experiences of changes in family systems were equivalent to a migration, the reasons for which, however, remained hidden from him at first. In the adoptive family, he grew up as an only child in an educationally deprived environment. Good performance at primary school initially helped him to grow into the family. Attending grammar school subsequently contributed more and more to alienation because knowledge and education contrasted with his adoptive parents' ideological attitudes. In the context of puberty, there were more outbursts of violence on the part of the father, whose role it was to translate the threat set up by the mother into physical humiliation. Niko was seeking 'an external stability without which he may go mad' (Winnicott et al. 2012/1984, p. 99). He openly asked the neighbour if she could be his mother, and he also felt closer to his friends' parents than to his adoptive family. In this uncertain terrain, he began to feel more and more like an 'outsider' who internalised as a flaw the rejection of the adoptive parents, which resulted in persistent avoidance of contact after he left his parents' home. The persistent confrontation with concrete issues was helpful for his personal development: playing the guitar (to find peace), martial arts (to compete with men in sports), political engagement (to rebel against authority and to channel his own anger) and studying education. The choice of topic for his thesis fell on adoption, especially since it was at this time that he first started a family of his own and became the father of a son for the first time, followed five years later by a second. Based on the assumption that the child's right to its own history should be central, the dissertation discussed the advantages and disadvantages of forms of adoption that were open to different degrees. From his own painful experience, he professionally advocated that the adopted child be effectively supported in his search for his own identity (Bittner 1992). His subsequent work as a social educator in youth services, where aggression was a recurring theme, allowed him to translate his own experiences into teaching, giving him direct access to children and young people, particularly those with problems, and to deal with their displays of aggression (Bittner 2000; Sickinger et al. 2008). He placed the topics of physicality, aggression and self-assertion in the context of youth-related identity development and was involved in the professional politics of the 'Landesarbeitsgemeinschaft Jungenarbeit Baden-Württemberg'. His professional development led to the implementation of self-defence training (also for women) and to trainer activities in the field of conflict management in adult education. As a school social worker, dealing with aggression shapes his everyday life on different levels: in preventive school and class actions, dispute mediator training and direct conflict regulation. As a Gestalt therapist who is familiar with creative methods (dance, martial arts, stick fighting, play), his attitude is oriented towards shaping contact and is characterised by a process-oriented approach.

Up to here, the authors' differences are very clear: Leticia, a foreign psychologist with an ontological-psychoanalytic background and coming from a collectivist culture, and Niko, a native educator and martial arts teacher with a background in Gestalt therapy connected to the approach of 'creative aggression' and coming from an individualistic culture.

2 A daunting challenge became the source of inspiration for the authors

From the perspective of leading a group, the authors clearly share markedly different foundation matrixes. For instance, they hold distinct mother tongues (both literally and metaphorically), were embedded in different cultures, and hold distinct genders – a major source of trouble for the foundation matrix (Foulkes and Foulkes 1990, pp. 152–153) and for conducting a group. On the level of the personal matrix, however, the two biographies reveal remarkable similarities: both are skilled foreigners and are migrants to differing degrees, both have experienced violence as part of their upbringing, both have lived through the feeling of being an 'outsider' in their own family, both have experienced deprivation, and both have overcome painful experiences and in line with Bohoslavsky (1998) have incorporated them constructively into their career choices.

The source of their desire to work with vulnerable children was in fact rooted in their personal matrixes. Owing to this personal matrix, they both developed unique skills in handling expressions of aggression. Hence, as outlined in chapter 1, both were (are) well-qualified for working with children with antisocial tendencies.

3 Some personal observations

What initially appeared to be a major obstacle to starting a group work with vulnerable children, namely the authors' diverse basic matrixes, has turned out to be a source of inspiration for the development of the fundamental means of T-WAS, namely the concept of the 'eclectic group conductors', which will be outlined in detail in chapter 5. To embrace diversity as a constructive matter has been of essential significance for the successful group work with vulnerable children as will be outlined further in chapters 8 and 9.

References

Bion, W.R., 1965. *Transformations: Change from Learning to Growth*. London: William Heinemann Medical Books.
Bion, W.R., 1984. *Attention & Interpretation*. London: Maresfield Reprints.
Bittner, N., 1992. *Sozialpädagogische Problem bei der Vermittlung von Fremdadoptionen. Zur Entwicklung und Diskussion offener Adoptionsformen*. Diplomarbeit: Universität Tübingen.
Bittner, N., 2000. *Selbstverteidigung für Jungen:. ein Trainingskonzept für Selbstverteidigungskurse mit Jungen*. Unpublished manuscript.
Blankertz, S., and Doubrawa, E., 2017. *Lexikon der Gestalttherapie*. Norderstedt: Books on Demand.
Bohoslavsky, R., 1998. *Orientación vocacional. La estratega clínica*. 20th ed. Buenos Aires: Nueva Visión.

Casement, P., 1991. *Learning from the Patient.* New York, London: Guilford Press.

Castrechini-Franieck, L., ed., 2022. *Communication with Vulnerable Patients: A Novel Psychological Approach.* London: Routledge.

Castrechini-Franieck, M.L., 2017. Wohin gehöre ich eigentlich? *JuKiP – Ihr Fachmagazin für Gesundheits- und Kinderkrankenpflege,* 6 (1), 36–39.

Castrechini-Franieck, M.L., Günter, M., and Page, T., 2014. Engaging Brazilian street children in play: Observations of their family narratives. *Child Development Research,* 2014, 861703.

Castrechini-Franieck, M.L., and Page, T., 2017. The family narratives of three siblings living in a 'street situation' since birth. *Early Child Development and Care,* 189 (10), 1575–1587.

Foulkes, S.H., and Foulkes, E., 1990. *Selected Papers of S.H. Foulkes: Psychoanalysis and Group Analysis.* Edited and with a brief biography by E. Foulkes. London: Karnac Books.

Franieck, L., and Günter, M., 2010. *On Latency: Individual Development, Narcissistic Impulse Reminiscence and Cultural Ideal.* London: Routledge.

Mann, D., 2020. *Gestalt Therapy: 100 Key Points & Techniques.* 2nd ed. London: Routledge.

Perls, F.S., Hefferline, R., and Goodman, P., 1994. *Gestalt Therapy: Excitement and Growth in the Human Personality.* Highland, NY: Gestalt Journal Press.

Sickinger, H., Bittner, N., Jerg, J., and Neubauer, G., 2008. *Jungenarbeit angemessen. Berichte, Anregungen, Materialien und Erkenntnisse aus einem Projekt für Jungen mit und ohne Assistenzbedarf.* Reutlingen: Diakonieverlag.

Winnicott, D.W., *et al.,* eds., 2012/1984. *Deprivation and Delinquency.* Abingdon: Routledge.

Chapter 5

'Eclectic group conductors'

I Eclectic group conductors – a novel means of leading children's groups

Castrechini-Franieck and Bittner (2022) asserted that like all vulnerable children, refugee children experience a continuous inner struggle against ambivalent values, as they are often confronted with contradictory realities. While some of the children can grow emotionally from this and learn to react flexibly to paradoxical situations (Hauser et al., 2006), others subsequently struggle with adjustment problems in social behaviour. They then remain stuck in their dilemmas, and experience them as painful, as being torn between two poles (like the complex interplay between aggression and love experienced by the infant, as mentioned in chapter 1) – a struggle that evokes 'either-or' thinking. The idea of 'shared meaning communication' (Castrechini-Franieck 2022) comes into play here when it regards differences less as dilemmas and more as choices that can be processed through 'both-as-also' thinking.

As ambiguous and paradoxical situations strongly affect vulnerable children's lives, particularly refugee children, this is precisely where they need support. The eclectic group conductors can model, initiate and repeatedly take up this 'shared meaning communication'. In this way, it is possible to support the children in achieving their emotional balance (homeostasis according to Gestalt), thus strengthening their resilience.

Castrechini-Franieck and Bittner (2022, p. 163) explained this as follows:

> 'Eclectic group conductors' can be perceived as a new approach in group work that intentionally uses the interplay of personal differences while conducting a group and putting the conductors' skills into action. This is more about using a resource in a relaxed and child-friendly way than worrying about the group conductor's own abilities to act, or whether their authority will be challenged... And it is also the idea that the quality of the relationship with the children is endangered if they come into contact with contradictions, as if this would weaken their trust in the group's leadership. At this point, it becomes clear that the way the

DOI: 10.4324/9781003466857-8

eclectic group conductors deal with contradictions is closely observed by the children and has a decisive influence on how the children get an idea of how to deal with ambiguities. The basis for this is our own certainty that we can actually offer the children corrective attachment experiences. The focus is not only on the relationship between the children and the conductors but more importantly on how the group conductors interact with each other. Both should work together in moderating the group and show a form of object relationship that includes an appreciative handling of the differences. Then there is a tangible offer to make both socially relevant experiences of parental representations and 'shared meaning communication', which has an encouraging effect on the children and stimulates them in their own development.

Achieving 'shared meaning communication' requires developing and sharing a common language with one another, between the eclectic group conductors and the children. As stated in the introduction, the common language adopted was the creative play that will be explained in more detail in chapter 7.

2 Eclectic group conductors and their mechanism

So far, particular emphasis has been laid on the eclectic group conductors as a resource for experiencing diversity. Hereafter, close attention will be given to the mechanisms and practices involved behind it, besides revealing how these mechanisms and practices can support this resource. To illustrate, it is essential to introduce the eclectic group conductors as two different individuals and as a unity in tandem. Whereas the former reinforces the symbol of polarities/diversity/ambiguity, the latter encourages the symbol of confluence/integration/cohesion.

3 Are they a unit or two different individuals?

The children perceived the eclectic group conductors as two individuals and as a unit in tandem. If the eclectic group conductors successfully manage their differences (i.e., gender model equality, their different mother tongues), as well as speaking 'with one clear voice' (see example below), then their unity can be emphasised. Starting at the end and working backwards, as long as the eclectic group conductors are aware of their differences and in spite of them are able to trust each other, a sense of unity can be passed on. Such unity, if understood in this way, allows space to perceive two individuals at once. Hence, a dilemma, an 'either-or' situation, is not encouraged, and diversity can be positively experienced and further assimilated (Castrechini-Franieck and Bittner 2022, pp. 161–163). Thus, the presence of both eclectic group conductors at all meetings was conceptually foreseen. If either of them was unable to attend, the group meeting was called off. A good example of diversity and the group conductors' coordination can be related to Leticia's challenges with the German language – a very similar situation to that experienced by children in children's homes in relation to their parents. Niko supported Leticia by patiently helping her to improve her language skills when it was necessary. It also happened that children laughed at Leticia's accent, and Niko then stood by Leticia by sorting out the children's behaviour and asking them for their understanding, whereupon the children apologised.

Two other ordinary situations that reflected how the children experienced the group conductors as belonging together – either as a unit or as two different individuals – were: 1) Every time when Leticia met one (or more than one) of the children outside the group setting (usually either on the street or on the aisle of the refugee camp), they immediately asked 'where is Niko?' 2) When Niko was unable to understand a child's remark, the child asked Leticia to 'translate' it for Niko. Figure 5.1 illustrates the potential interactions between the eclectic group conductors and the children.

4 Backstage work

For eclectic group conductors to manage and carefully integrate diversity, they need to raise awareness of the co-existing external and internal variables that may influence their performance, a point that Westman (1996) stresses but does not elaborate on. The variables we referred to are presented in Figure 5.2.

The eclectic group conductors hold different roles in tandem that may be interchangeably experienced while leading the group, that is, as group conductors, as qualified professional colleagues, as internal/external employees of an organisation and as private people. As group conductors, they should focus on mutual appreciation, harmony and good partnership. As qualified

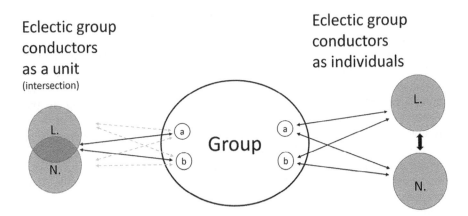

Figure 5.1 Eclectic group conductors reference points.

Internal Influences   External Influences

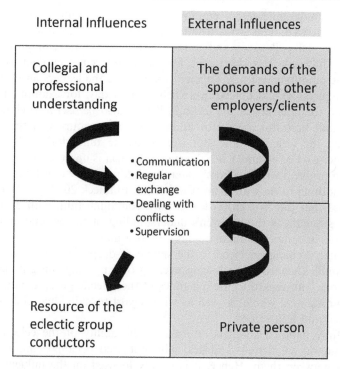

Figure 5.2 Eclectic group conductors roles.

professional colleagues, they should establish a sense of mutual security, trust, friendship, honesty and mutual respect. As internal/external employees of an organisation, they are in charge of their tasks, schedules, decision making, time keeping, ability to deal with stressful situations and any political issues. As private people, they are linked to and are affected by family and/or personal problems, past emotional experiences and their own personality. Continuous clarification of these roles is crucial, not only to support them as resources, but also to broaden their understanding of the group matrix (Foulkes, 2018a; 2018b). Otherwise, a potential conflict area might emerge (see chapter 9, transcript 1). With the aim of achieving this clarification, the authors adopted four basic procedures: 1) mutual understanding communication, 2) regular professional exchange, 3) conscious handling of conflicts and 4) supervision, which are illustrated below.

1   Communication in the field of mutual understanding involved an agreement to meet a few minutes before the group session to allow time for a chat or for an emotional settling in. If feelings of anger or frustration remained due to demands from another field of work or due to personal issues, these could be discussed. In this way, it is possible to clarify the

roles as internal/external employees of an organisation and as private people as well. This leads to an improvement in their roles as qualified professional colleagues and a mutual understanding can grow. Sometimes, however, this short time for discussion is not enough to process strong emotions; yet it is sufficient for making the leaders aware that the colleague(s) should not be overwhelmed that day, for example. Depending on the intensity of the feelings, it may also be useful to clarify whether and how this should be addressed in the group with the children during the welcome time slot (see 'welcome time slot' explanation in chapter 6). For example, if Niko states, 'Leticia is upset today because she had a problem with her boss', then the children know that Leticia's mood has nothing to do with them (Castrechini-Franieck 2022, p. 79) and they realise that the two group leaders are communicating with each other. This strengthens the children's understanding of the eclectic group conductors as tangible human beings and as a unit.

2   Regular exchange referred to the sphere of deepening the qualified professional knowledge. Following every group meeting, insights and evaluations with regard to the dynamics of the eclectic group conductors, of the group as a whole, as well as with regard to individual children were shared and transcribed.

3   Skilfully handled conflicts referred to the ability of the eclectic group conductors to identify and deal with potential personal emotional conflicts between them. Hence, it is mostly focused on the influence of the private person role. Once, a German reporter wanted to write an article about the children's group. The responsibility for obtaining photo consent was disputed by Leticia and the reporter. This unresolved impasse led to upset between the two during the course of the report. The reporter addressed her questions almost exclusively to Niko and avoided contact with Leticia. This frustration led to a verbal exchange of blows between Letica and Niko afterwards, as Leticia felt highly irritated. In her private person sphere, being left out of the interview initially resulted in anger, as this was a situation Leticia had experienced multiple times in Germany – being ignored because she was a foreigner. At that moment, Niko became for her one more member of this German group (society). Leticia simply projected her difficult experiences onto Niko, especially as Niko had done nothing to change the situation in the course of the interview. Leticia's courage in revealing her personal vulnerability in this mutual handling of conflicts occasioned a deeper insight into their view of group leadership. Additionally, a representation could be given to her feelings via a container-contained process (Bion 1984a; 1984b) and via a 'mutuality' process (Winnicott 2018). Leticia and Niko realised that the feelings of impotence aroused in Leticia were probably very similar to the ones we presumed the children and their parents were familiar with – countertransference matters as outlined by Ballhausen-Scharf et al. (2021);

Trautmann-Voigt and Voigt (2019); Westman (1996); Haar and Wenzel (2019); Foulkes and Anthony (1990).

4   Regarding the supervision, this was attended privately and individually by both Leticia and Niko, to clarify their own understanding of their roles and for further connection with their private emotional worlds.

5 Some essential requirements on leading a children's group

Leading a group of children involves fulfilling some basic requirements, which can ensure the creation of a secure and protected space for the children (a 'holding' environment in Winnicott's terms (1960)). Among them, three are essential, namely: 1) the group conductors' clear awareness of their role as the ideal parental representation (Slavson 1950; Slavson and Schiffer 1975; Westman 1996); 2) the playful abilities of the group conductors, combined with the expression of their genuine desire to make contact with the children (Foulkes and Anthony 1990; Lehle 2018; Moll 1997; Slavson 1950; Slavson and Schiffer 1975) and 3) the mutual determination to maintain the group structure (Bach and Goldberg 1976; Blom 2006; Franck 1997; Winnicott et al. 2012/1984; Woods 1993). These three conditions are discussed in more detail below.

5.1 Awareness of the role of parental representation

In general, it is expected that the children will transfer their ideal mother/ father representations onto the group conductors (Slavson 1950; Westman 1996). However, the group conductors need to be aware that leading new experiences of family-like communication does not imply identifying themselves with these projections. On the contrary, it involves a similar process to the 'maternal reverie' (Bion 1984a) in which these projections should be grasped, processed and given back to the children by the group conductors with the clarity that they are not their actual mother and/or father (Blom 2006; Oaklander 2001). An ordinary and concrete example is that when cooking together, a child may say, 'Leticia, my mum does it like this!' to which Leticia would reply, 'Really? Thanks for showing me, but don't forget, this is Leticia's way now!' Other situations may happen on a more counter-transferential level as emphasised by Foulkes and Anthony (1990) and that is why it is important to keep the four basic practices as previously described.

5.2 Play skills

This brings us to the second professional requirement for eclectic group conductors. This is expressed in the self-image of one's own curiosity and joy found in play – the ability to enact. Entering into the communication field of play serves as a space opener for coming into contact with the child in the child's world and for grasping the relationship to each other and with each other in its manifold variations whilst trying out the relationship in an imaginative way (Slavson and Schiffer 1975; Foulkes and Anthony 1990). This also includes encouraging ideas that are initially regarded as 'crazy', such as the 'excrement machine' (in childish language 'poo machine'), to be played out in the group (see description of the game in chapter 7). Playfulness occurs when one is familiar with one's own inner child, and is able to feel whole, even when the acquired attributes of the adult world are absent. To this end, the eclectic group conductors may be a model for the children for the ways in which adults can be affectionate towards them. For example, Niko, like many children before him, was glued to the wall after he won a card game and requested this (see Figure 5.3).

Of course, while playing with the children, no one actually becomes a child. We remained present, as this is needed to maintain elementary boundaries and to preserve the group's structure. Closeness builds a bond that also has an effect on the children's willingness to accept rules from the eclectic group conductors in the game, as well as in the group as a whole.

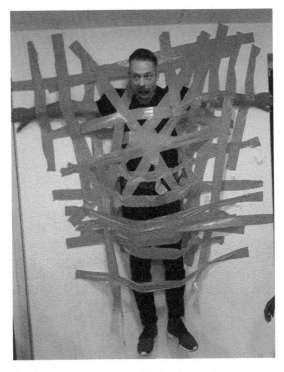

Figure 5.3 Niko glued.
Source: From Figure 8.2: 'Glued to the wall', p. 173, *Communicating with Vulnerable Patients: A Novel Psychological Approach*, by Maria Leticia Castrechini Fernandes Franieck, © 2023 by Imprint. Reproduced by Routledge, permission of Taylor & Francis Group.

5.3 Holding up group structure

This brings us to the third basic prerequisite for group work with children – the common will to maintain the group's structure without becoming tyrannical (Woods 1993). The ability to set limits and rules without fear of possible angry/aggressive reactions from the children means getting in touch with one's own aggressive impulses – the basic aspect of constructive aggression according to Bach and Goldberg (1976). Hence, the 'rule check' was regarded as one of the important leading tasks of the eclectic group conductors.

5.3.1 Rule check

Basically, a list of rules was created and written down on a flipchart together with the children. Agreeing on common rules was an important point for developing a secure room and at the same time an understanding of the group. In this sense, the rule check was an ongoing process of regulating social interaction, particularly in an open group setting with an undefined group size, as was the case with T-WAS. This led to new situations whenever new group members came along, so that the 'veterans' were able to explain the rules to the 'new' children. Hence, gradually, both a sense of responsibility (Blom 2006), as well as the development of the capacity for concern (Winnicott et al. 2012/1984) might emerge.

At every group session, the paper from the flipchart was hung up and was thus a reference point for compliance with the process of rules over and over again. Lots of rules were suggested by the children themselves, such as the 14th rule. The rules were: 1) speak only German, 2) do not insult others, 3) do not spit, 4) do not hit others, 5) do not yell/shout, 6) no physical altercations, 7) be punctual, 8) do not threaten others, 9) no mobile phones or personal toys, 10) no eating, drinking or chewing gum, 11) anyone who breaks the rules will receive a warning, 12) after three warnings, the person in question must leave the group (is excluded), 13) anyone who comes to the group must stay until the end, 14) listen to Leticia and Niko.

For rules 11 and 12, which led to warnings and/or expulsion from the group, according to the case in question, there was the need for further clarification, which was addressed via a personal conversation. The goal was to trigger reflection on the conflict that had arisen while practising positive aggression. At the same time, we also felt it important to value the child's need for further participation, understood as a desire to accept their aggressive energy (Blom 2006) or primary aggression (Winnicott, 2014/1945). We allowed the child to feel that his/her aggressive energy / primary aggression had been absorbed by us. When the conflict was intense, the clarifying talk usually took place alongside the group session. Generally, this led to the male group leader dealing with the boys and the female group leader dealing with the girls, or both of them together when the conflict was really intense. If the latter was the case, then an extra, short, individual session was arranged.

If the group is larger (more than 12 children), it must be made clear from the outset that, due to the size of the group, only one warning will be given for breaking the rules. A second means leaving the group.

6 Some personal observations

So far, the presence of diversity in group work, especially with children, has been treated as background noise that is mostly ignored or even 'interpreted' as potentially disruptive. In fact, the idea of safety has been mistaken for the idea of being free from disruption, like being in Nirvana – a utopia. The healthiest security that one person can offer to another consists of being by their side during the course of disruptive experiences – metaphorically speaking, being a safe harbour, no matter how stormy the sea may be. In our opinion, it is worth keeping one's ears open to this disturbing background noise because once it is there, it is part of the context and should definitely not be ignored. At the very core of our reflection on the meaning of eclectic group conductors lies the attitude towards diversity.

References

Bach, G.R., and Goldberg, H., 1976. *Creative Aggression*. London: Coventure.

Ballhausen-Scharf, B., *et al.*, 2021. *Gruppenanalyse mit Kindern und Jugendlichen. Ein Leitfaden zur Kompetenzentwicklung*. Goettingen: Vandenhoeck & Ruprecht.

Bion, W.R., 1984a. *Learning from Experience*. London: Maresfield.

Bion, W.R., 1984b. *Second Thoughts: Selected Papers on Psychoanalysis*. London: Routledge.

Blom, R., 2006. *The Handbook of Gestalt Play Therapy: Practical Guidelines for Child Therapists*. London: Jessica Kingsley Publishers.

Castrechini-Franieck, L., ed., 2022. *Communication with Vulnerable Patients: A Novel Psychological Approach*. London: Routledge.

Castrechini-Franieck, L., and Bittner, N., 2022. T-WAS: Together We Are Strong. In L. Castrechini-Franieck (ed.), *Communication with Vulnerable Patients: A Novel Psychological Approach*. London: Routledge, 155–185.

Foulkes, S.H., 2018a. *Group-Analytic Psychotherapy: Method and Principles*. London: Routledge.

Foulkes, S.H., 2018b. *Therapeutic Group Analysis*. London: Routledge.

Foulkes, S.H., and Anthony, E.J., 1990. *Group Psychotherapy: The Psychoanalytic Approach*. 2nd ed. London: Routledge.

Franck, J., 1997. *Gestalt-Gruppentherapie mit Kindern*. 1st ed. Freiamt: Arbor-Verl.

Haar, R., and Wenzel, H., 2019. *Psychodynamische Gruppentherapie mit Kindern*. 1st ed. Stuttgart: Kohlhammer.

Hauser, S.T., Allen, J.P., and Golden, E., 2006. *Out of the Woods: Tales of Resilient Teens*. . Cambridge, MA, London: Harvard University Press.

Lehle, H.G., 2018. 'Egotraining in Aktion'. Das Spiel in der psychoanalytischen Kindergruppentherapie. In B. Traxl, ed. *Psychodynamik im Spiel. Psychoanalytische*

Überlegungen und klinische Erfahrungen zur Bedeutung des Spiels. Frankfurt AM: Brandes & Apsel, 133–158.

Moll, M., 1997. Thesen zur gruppenanalytischen Arbeit mit Kindern. *Arbeitshefte Gruppenanalyse*, 12, 22–31.

Oaklander, V., 2001. Gestalt play therapy. *International Journal of Play Therapy*, 10 (2), 45–55.

Slavson, S.R., 1950. *Analytic Group Psychotherapy: With Children Adolescents and Adults.* New York: Columbia University Press.

Slavson, S.R., and Schiffer, M., 1975. *Group Psychotherapies for Children: A Textbook.* New York: International Universities Press.

Trautmann-Voigt, S., and Voigt, B., eds., 2019. *Mut zur Gruppentherapie! Das Praxisbuch für gruppenaffine Psychotherapeuten: Leitfäden Interventionstipps Antragsbeispiele nach der neuen PT-Richtlinie.* Stuttgart: Schattauer.

Westman, A., 1996. Cotherapy and 're-parenting' in a group for disturbed children. *Group Analysis*, 29 (1), 55–68.

Winnicott, D.W., 1960. The theory of the parent-child relationship. *International Journal of Psycho-Analysis*, 41, 585–595.

Winnicott, D.W., 2014/1945. Aggression in relation to emotional development. In D. W. Winnicott (ed.), *Collected Papers: Through Paediatrics to Psycho-Analysis.* London: Routledge, 204–218.

Winnicott, D.W., et al., eds., 2012/1984. *Deprivation and Delinquency.* Abingdon: Routledge.

Winnicott, D.W., 2018. The mother-infant experience of mutuality. In *Psycho-Analytic Explorations.* London: Routledge, 251–260.

Woods, J., 1993. Limits and structure in child group psychotherapy. *Journal of Child Psychotherapy*, 19 (1), 63–78.

Chapter 6

Settings

The structural setting of T-WAS embodies four pillars, three phases, a temporal structure of a group meeting divided into three timeslots and finally its basic shape and boundary lines.

I The pillars of T-WAS

T-WAS consists of four basic methodological pillars. These are described below and illustrated in Figure 6.1.

1   Eclectic group conductors is the central pillar as referred to in chapter 5.
2   Anger management can be perceived as supervised and regulated cathartic play/games that seek to discharge the group's non-symbolic anger, or 'the aggressive energy' as termed by Blom (2006), Oaklander (1988) and Franck (1997). The play session/games are divided into ritualised and non-ritualised activities. The former belongs to the time structure of the group meeting; the latter are optional and may be adopted if the group is restless after the 'starting ritual' (further details are provided in chapter 7).
3   Ego-strengthening (ego-relatedness experiences) can be improved via in-group experiences or via 'ego training in action', as termed by Foulkes and Anthony (1990) with regards to three different dimensions: a) by playing games that promote cooperative skills, i.e., team spirit, focusing on experiencing and processing group dynamics; b) engaging the imagination to expand children's representation and verbal expression of more shameful issues in a safe environment; and c) through family-like experiences – as the name suggests, 'ego-relatedness' experiences are those that correspond to the ones within the family (Moll 1997). Full details of all games are provided in chapter 7.
4   Reflection happens in two distinct moments: a) during the group meeting, together with the children, when the children express their thoughts about their experiences within the group (more details are supplied later in this chapter); and b) after the group meeting, when written transcriptions of the group sessions are made, and the eclectic group conductors share their impressions and perceptions of their roles and/or conflict situations

DOI: 10.4324/9781003466857-9

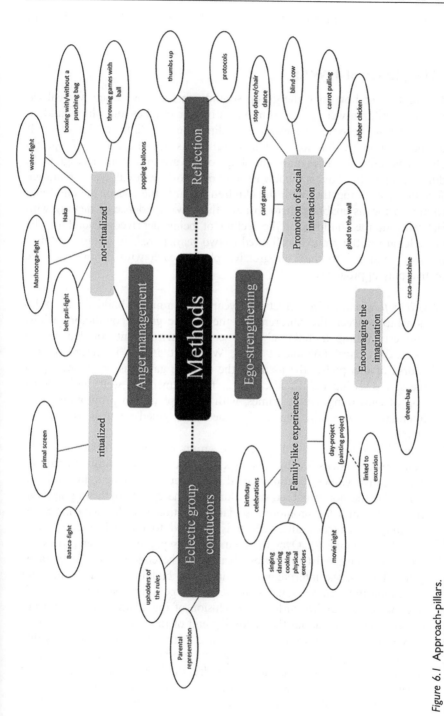

Figure 6.1 Approach-pillars.

in the group (Ballhausen-Scharf et al. 2021; Cividini-Strani and Klain 1984; Hofmann 2010; Westman 1996).

2 The phases of T-WAS

The question of how long the group should run for arose when we realised that some children were going to move with their families and older children were going to become teenagers, exceeding the age limit of 13 years. It became clear to us that we wanted to actively shape the end of the group before these circumstances made the shape of the group no longer tangible. In addition, separation/loss is the key issue in our work with vulnerable children. Working actively together with the children towards the end of the children's group also means enabling them to have the new experience of dealing with grief without the shadows of the feeling of being deprived. Therefore, the course length of the group was limited to two years (circa. 70 group meetings) and was divided into three progressive phases, each with its own specific creative play approaches:

1   *Group formation phase* (first half year): this aims to build up the relationship between the children and the eclectic group conductors, whilst also establishing a 'holding' (and secure) environment coupled with a 'potential space' (Winnicott 1953; Winnicott 1960). Therefore, in the course of this phase, the focus of the creative games is on the set-up of the group setting via ritualised anger management, as well the introduction of ego-strengthening games, with an emphasis on promoting social interaction, especially the card games and 'glued to wall' (details in chapter 7).
2   *Consolidation phase* (a full year): the group structure consolidates. Relationships are intensified by new experiences of the self within the group. The creative games remain focused on anger management methods, in particular the non-ritualised one, alongside the ego-strengthening approaches. All games for promoting social interaction may be played, besides birthdays being celebrated, which is assigned to family-like experiences (details in chapter 7). Over the course of this phase, a deeper process of reflection connected to the strengthening of the children's resilience takes place. That is, the interpretation training for building a 'shared meaning communication' makes the first move in this period (Castrechini-Franieck and Bittner 2022). Towards the conclusion of this phase, the children are carefully informed about the upcoming end of the group.
3   *Farewell phase* (last six months): dealing with and coping with possible ambivalent experiences (e.g., separation, gender roles, different cultures and cultural ideals) is increasingly addressed in this phase. Besides the creative games mentioned previously, more family-like experiences and the promotion of imagination should now be in the foreground to

support the thinking that ambiguities should be seen less as dilemmas and more as choices that can be processed/managed through 'both... as well as...' – that is to support the achievement of the 'shared meaning communication'.

3 Time structure of a group meeting

Each group meeting lasted 90 minutes and was appointed on the same weekday, at the same time of day, and in the same biggest communal room of the shared housing for refugees. Ordinarily, the time structure of a group meeting is compiled of three timeslots: the *welcome timeslot*, the *play timeslot* and the *closing timeslot*.

The *welcome timeslot* is mostly focused on the first encounter with the children. The children arrive and are greeted by the eclectic group conductors with a 'hello' or a high-five or even a hug when this gesture comes from the children themselves. A casual and ordinary chat starts, as is common in a family, whilst the chairs are put altogether in a circle. Afterwards, the names of the children are written on a name badge. Group rules are recalled and are displayed on the flip chart. If there is a special feature to be announced that concerns today's group activities, this is the time for that. Through these short chats, initial impressions about the emotional state of each child 'here and now' (Perls et al. 1994; Riesenberg-Malcolm 1999) can be gained. The level of the children's excitement can be sensed.

Playtime slot begins with a starting ritual – the 'bataca-fight' (a cathartic activity that is overseen and regulated) – that enables (and contains) the collective release of any previous anger in the group (Blom 2006; Haar and Wenzel 2019; Hofmann 2019; Lucas 1988). The release of aggressive energy must first be processed through playfulness, so that the expression of emotion can flow spontaneously (Blom 2006, pp. 119–123). The next step is to pose the question: 'And what do we play now?' At this point, the children can easily engage in the creative games, and they are free to choose what they want to play. If there is a consensus on what to play, then this game is played. If not, then the card game (see description in chapter 7) arose as a favourite means of establishing a winner (or, rarely, more than one winner) by chance, who would then be allowed to decide what the group would play together. In this way, the winner has the opportunity to gain experience of performing the role of group leader while building their self-confidence within the group.

The last 10–15 minutes of the group meeting is dedicated to the *farewell timeslot*, which includes a reflection combined with a 'closing ritual'. Here is also the time for recalling important information that was shared during the welcome timeslot. The reflection is triggered each time by the same question: 'How was the group today?' The children express their assessment non-verbally with their thumbs. Thumbs up means 'good' or 'approval', thumbs across/horizontal means 'so so' or 'satisfactory' and thumbs down stands for 'bad' or 'disapproval'. This gives everyone a chance to express their feelings about how the group is doing, considering the fluctuation in group size. The eclectic group conductors usually give their feedback at the end to summarise and conclude any disagreements that may have arisen during the reflection time (Castrechini-Franieck 2022, p. 47). Lastly, there is a closing ritual represented by the 'primal scream' (Casriel 1972) – a regulated cathartic expression of all the frustration experienced during the group session. The group stand in a circle; everyone holds hands, counts to three and shouts 'haaaaa' together. Then, the chairs are cleared away and goodbyes are said, individually if some children are still seeking contact.

On special occasions, such as movie evenings, Olympiad, Christmas celebrations, outings or projects, this time structure is disrupted. Regarding the starting and closing rituals, both are described in more detail in chapter 7.

4 Basic shape and boundary lines

At the start, when the group was being formed, there were no assessments – prior biographical information about neither the children nor their family was gathered. Rather, there was evidence of a chaotic environment in the shared housing for refugees, such as cultural and family disruptions, vandalism and walls painted with many scrawled sexual symbols and innuendos. The religious sponsors were overwhelmed by this messy situation. T-WAS was introduced directly to the children as a free-will, low-threshold offering and it was promoted verbally by the social workers working in the shared housing for refugees and also by posters put up on the walls of the shared housing for refugees. The groups were open, i.e., new members could join at any time, which meant that the group could vary in size greatly – from three (although rarely) up to 24 children. In fact, the children were supposed to join the group of their own free will – the natural means for promoting 'moment of meeting' (Stern et al. 1998). The target group was children from six up to 13 years old from different cultural backgrounds, mostly from Afghanistan, Africa, Syria, Iraq and Iran. We realised that the age difference very rarely posed an obstacle for our target group, especially if siblings stayed together as they helped to give the group structure. Hence, we formed two gender-separated groups, with each group meeting fortnightly. However, once a month, during birthday celebrations (see description of the birthday celebration in chapter 7), both groups were together for circa 15 minutes. Nonetheless, the children could change the group to a mixed-gender group themselves if everyone aimed to meet weekly (more details in chapter 8). The standard equipment and tools available in a group children's therapy room, such as dolls, drawing and/or painting utensils and/or writing boards, as well as movement-oriented materials, were not available in the communal room of the shared housing for refugees. Rather, creative games mostly focused on promoting team and family orientation were adopted, as described in chapter 7.

The initial approach was the presence of the eclectic group conductor in the communal room, waiting for the children whilst not knowing how many of them would come, nor what games exactly would be played, nor what kind of conflicts would be dealt with. Put simply, the group conductor was waiting without any desire in the sense emphasised by Bion (1984), while ready for initiating a new group matrix as raised by Foulkes (2018a; 2018b; Foulkes and Foulkes 1990).

As previously mentioned, setting boundaries in group work with children, according to Ginott (1979), is a controversial topic, as it is connected to different ways of defining 'allowing'. For instance, Foulkes and Anthony (1990) suggested setting as few limits as possible. Lehle (2018) recommended a setting that provides support and safety with clearly defined rules and agreements. Blom (2006) understood boundaries and limitations as essential since they provide structure and security for the child, and Woods (1993) emphasised the care that must be taken when setting limits so that they do not turn into an expression or an acting out of the group leader (otherwise they can trigger anxiety in the members of the group).

In view of T-WAS-specific points, structured boundaries were to be implemented to support in-group relationships, as well as to guide the children on not crossing the line. Hence, T-WAS pursues the following four main tenets:

1   The children can refer to the conductors by calling them by their first names, Leticia and Niko, as using an informal form of 'you' in German language. The aim is to achieve 'two-way communication' with the children or a basic dialogical attitude, like in Gestalt therapy, on an equal level.
2   All decisions concerning the group should be made democratically, with room for discussion and the exchanging of ideas (the same aim as before). The role of the eclectic group conductors is to present different points of view for discussion, encouraging the children to reflect and to practise 'shared meaning communication'.
3   All group members follow the 14 basic rules described in chapter 5.
4   The children should take on a number of tasks for the organisation of the group, such as setting up the chairs in a circle in the room before the group starts and putting the chairs back at the end of the group.

5 Some personal observations

Similar to the Transient Interactive Communication Approach or TICA (Castrechini-Franieck 2022), T-WAS can also be perceived as a novel approach, due to its peculiar features, when compared to other forms of psychosocial group work. Its pillars cover Gestalt (i.e., anger management) and ontological psychoanalysis (i.e., ego-relatedness experiences) theoretical backgrounds. Its phases were basically focused on in-group relationship development – most of the creative games adopted come from Gestalt therapy and the pedagogical field; however the features of relatedness triggered by them are conceived with ontological psychoanalysis in mind. The time structure of the meeting is well defined by the presence of starting and closing rituals, which in their turn improve the children's ability to gain a clear sense of time and of meaning, alongside a kind of 'holding' as referred to in chapter 2. Regarding the basic format, one of the major challenges was the high fluctuation of the group size, as the group has an open character. According to Foulkes (2018b, p. 40), open groups tend to be more individual-centred and more leader-centred. In the case of T-WAS, the aim is not only to focus on the eclectic group conductors as a reference point for the children, but above all to create a milieu susceptible to diversities. In other words, as long as new members can join the group at any time, the likelihood that the participating children will have to deal with more diversity and ambiguity naturally increases. Undoubtedly this means that the eclectic group conductors should be able to deal with diversities and ambiguities without losing themselves.

References

Ballhausen-Scharf, B., *et al.*, 2021. *Gruppenanalyse mit Kindern und Jugendlichen. Ein Leitfaden zur Kompetenzentwicklung.* Goettingen: Vandenhoeck & Ruprecht.

Bion, W.R., 1984. *Attention & Interpretation.* London: Maresfield Reprints.

Blom, R., 2006. *The Handbook of Gestalt Play Therapy: Practical Guidelines for Child Therapists.* London: Jessica Kingsley Publishers.

Casriel, D., 1972. *A Scream Away from Happiness.* New York: Grosset & Dunlap.

Castrechini-Franieck, L., ed., 2022. *Communication with Vulnerable Patients: A Novel Psychological Approach.* London: Routledge.

Castrechini-Franieck, L., and Bittner, N., 2022. T-WAS: Together We Are Strong. In L. Castrechini-Franieck (ed.), *Communication with Vulnerable Patients: A Novel Psychological Approach.* London: Routledge, 155–185.

Cividini-Strani, E., and Klain, E., 1984. Advantages and disadvantages of co-therapy. *Group Analysis*, 17 (2), 156–159.

Foulkes, S.H., 2018a. *Group-Analytic Psychotherapy: Method and Principles.* London: Routledge.

Foulkes, S.H., 2018b. *Therapeutic Group Analysis.* London: Routledge.

Foulkes, S.H., and Anthony, E.J., 1990. *Group Psychotherapy. The Psychoanalytic Approach.* 2nd ed. London: Routledge.

Foulkes, S.H., and Foulkes, E., 1990. *Selected Papers of S.H. Foulkes: Psychoanalysis and Group Analysis.* Edited and with a brief biography by E. Foulkes. London: Karnac Books.

Franck, J., 1997. *Gestalt-Gruppentherapie mit Kindern.* 1st ed. Freiamt: Arbor-Verl.

Ginott, H.G., 1979. *Gruppenpsychotherapie mit Kindern. Theorie und Praxis der Spieltherapie.* Frankfurt am Main: Fischer.

Haar, R., and Wenzel, H., 2019. *Psychodynamische Gruppentherapie mit Kindern*. 1st ed. Stuttgart: Kohlhammer.

Hofmann, E., 2010. Gruppenanalytische Arbeit mit Kindern: Eine Gruppe wird 'geboren'. Stufen im Prozess zu einer ambulanten Kindergruppe. *Gruppenanalyse*, 20 (1), 53–81.

Hofmann, E., 2019. Nach-Denken über eine gestaltende Kinder- und Jugentlichengruppe in einem Erstaufnahmezentrum für Asylsuchende. *Gruppenanalyse*, 29 (1), 7–20.

Lehle, H.G., 2018. *Freiräume des Spiels. Psychoanalytische Gruppentherapie mit Kindern und Jugendlichen*. Frankfurt am Main: Brandes & Apsel.

Lucas, T., 1988. Holding and holding-on: Using Winnicott's ideas in group psychotherapy with twelve- to thirteen-year-olds. *Group Analysis*, 21 (2), 135–149.

Moll, M., 1997. Thesen zur gruppenanalytischen Arbeit mit Kindern. *Arbeitshefte Gruppenanalyse*, 12, 22–31.

Oaklander, V., 1988. *Windows to Our Children: A Gestalt Therapy Approach to Children and Adolescents*. Highland, NY: Center for Gestalt Development.

Perls, F.S., Hefferline, R., and Goodman, P., 1994. *Gestalt Therapy: Excitement and Growth in the Human Personality*. Highland, NY: Gestalt Journal Press.

Riesenberg-Malcolm, R., 1999. Interpretation: The past in the present. In P.L. Roth (ed.), *On Bearing Unbearable States of Mind*. London: Routledge, 38–52.

Stern, D.N., *et al.*, 1998. Non-interpretive mechanisms in psychoanalytic therapy: The 'something more' than interpretation. *The International Journal of Psychoanalysis*, 79 (5), 903–921.

Westman, A., 1996. Cotherapy and 're-parenting' in a group for disturbed children. *Group Analysis*, 29 (1), 55–68.

Winnicott, D.W., 1953. Transitional objects and transitional phenomena: A study of the first not-me possession. *International Journal of Psycho-Analysis*, 34, 89–97.

Winnicott, D.W., 1960. The theory of the parent-child relationship. *International Journal of Psycho-Analysis*, 41, 585–595.

Woods, J., 1993. Limits and structure in child group psychotherapy. *Journal of Child Psychotherapy*, 19 (1), 63–78.

Chapter 7

Creative play

As referred to in chapter 6, T-WAS is made up of four basic methodological pillars. In this chapter, the focus is on three of them, namely: anger management, ego-strengthening and reflection. The authors present in detail the manner in which they made use of the creative play to support communication among the group members whilst creating a playful/transitional space. In this secure environment, the children were able to re-experiment their id impulses (or primary aggression) and aggressive energy in a framework of ego-relatedness, improving, therefore, their resilience and achieving 'shared meaning communication'.

1 Ritualised anger management

1.1 Batacas 'fight' – the starting ritual

The bataca, also called the anti-aggression bat or anger club, is a common tool adopted by Gestalt therapy during the phase of the expression of aggressive energy (Blom, 2006; Oaklander, 1988). Despite all the controversy surrounding the Gestalt therapeutic thesis of the positive and therapeutic effects of aggression release (as with Batakas) – as opposed to the more dys-regulation-based theory (LeCroy, 1988) – we endorse Lucas' ideas (1988) referred to in chapter 3 that games should be introduced into group work with vulnerable children to create a 'safe space' in which children can act out their primary aggression and at the same time develop their associative thinking. However, in order to provide such a 'protected space' (Winnicott, 1960), the group conductor(s) must be able to tolerate and transform violent impulses. This is a crucial skill in leading groups with vulnerable children (Woods, 1996). This is particularly important when working with children with antisocial tendencies, as inner tensions do not yet have a conscious point of reference because of a lack of symbolisation caused by the deprivation (Winnicott et al., 2012/1984). In the context of T-WAS, aggression should be processed in-group, right at the beginning of a group session, as a common feeling, and when the eclectic group conductors played the bataca together

DOI: 10.4324/9781003466857-10

with the children, they connected the cathartic action with verbal expression of their feelings of anger. That is, they laid emphasis on the importance of translating activity and tension into words, as referred to by Oaklander (1988), as well as by Foulkes und Anthony (1990). It has also been used to transform sensory information or misrepresented/disorganised experience (beta elements) into creative thinking (alpha elements), providing the mind with a thinking apparatus, as outlined by Bion (1984a; 1984b). The aim of this starting ritual is to establish a constructive way of dealing with aggressive energy (and primary aggression) through a supervised form of fighting. This involves foam-covered sticks (with padded handles) that can be used to hit people without hurting anyone, similar to a pillow fight when the pillows are held by the corners. The batacas bats are available in two sizes; the small ones are well suited for children up to around ten years.

The fight procedure is precisely defined. Everyone sits in a circle. The group conductors communicate the fight's rules, such as the hitting area, the length of the fight and end-of-fight closing rituals (salutation). Then, a child is chosen at random to start the fight, i.e., one of the group conductors rotates blindfolded in the centre of the circle with an outstretched arm until the other group conductor says 'stop' and the child to whom the arm points may begin. This selection method was welcomed by the children. The chosen child first decides whether his/her successor will be the one on his/her right or left side. Then he/she invites another child in the circle to fight, who, by the way, may say 'yes' or 'no'. In a 'big round', which is adopted over the group formation phase, each child may challenge once, no matter how many times he or she has already been challenged, whereas in a 'small round', each child only fights once. The 'small round' is introduced from the consolidation phase onwards, after the 'big round' has been successfully established. Hence, at the beginning of each group, it is possible to ask the children whether they would like a 'small' or 'big' round. Concerning the fight's rules, the hitting area is the hip of the other person. Deviations upwards and downwards can be tolerated in the range of one hand-width each way. Intentional blows to the head and genitals were expressly forbidden, and if this happened the child was automatically expelled from the group session. Two children grab each other's forearms crosswise in the so-called 'lumberjack grip', i.e., the left hand grabs the left forearm of the other. Both children agree on who will start. Each child has two trial strokes, one of medium strength followed by a strong one. When both children agree to this strength of stroke, they can start. Then, the group conductors give the command 'On your mark, get set, go' and the children start hitting as hard as they can for ten seconds. The group conductors invite all children to count out loud to ten and then say: '*And STOP!*' By fighting together with batacas, aggression can be discharged with strength in a playful way and without hurting the other person. Encouraging all group members to count together out loud builds an animated neutral space that supports the release of aggression in a controlled way. In Oaklander's (1988;

2001) terms, this is also the mirror aspect of showing oneself to the other children in the group, of exposing oneself to everyone's gaze in the middle of the circle whilst fighting. If a left-handed person meets a right-handed person, they both first hold each other with their right hands for 5 seconds, then they switch and hold each other with their left hands for 5 seconds. Once the fight is over, the children should put down their batacas and proceed with the end-of-fight parting gestures. The latter can be described as a polite gesture via one last form of body contact, signifying respect and connection. Three different types of greetings are possible according to an ascending pattern of physical contact: 1) mutual touching of the little fingers, 2) high-fives with the palms of the hands, and 3) hugging. The type of body contact with the smaller body contact area has priority, e.g., if one child only wants to high-five, they do not have to let themselves be hugged. However, when the eclectic group conductors have a fight together, they end up hugging each other, which has a great positive emotional impact on the children.

Guidance notes: Having batacas of both sizes was appropriate for the fluctuating T-WAS age group, as it allowed all children to participate equally. Freewill with regards to participation in the fight is crucial; yet the idea of togetherness is often cultivated. If the group is larger (more than 12 children) and there are a lot of new members, it is advisable to do a 'small round' as some children may get annoyed if they have to wait their turn and start disturbing the group (illustration in chapter 9, transcription 3). Any type of biased expression (ethnic, cultural, religious or gender) due to diversities in which a group member is placed in a disadvantaged or excluded position should be accurately addressed by the group conductors, as the game is also about the uninhibited expression of aggression. The incentive is to create an equally transitional space for all, thus the fight may be conducted without restraint on either side (Bach & Goldberg, 1976). To illustrate, the size difference between the children can be resolved by asking the bigger child to kneel to be at the same height as the smaller child in order for there to be a fair fight. If the bigger child refuses to kneel (i.e., due to pride), then one of the group conductors will ask this child to return to his/her seat and then one of the group conductors will be the new bataca-partner for the smaller child. The same approach was adopted, either when a child had difficulties in getting in touch with his/her anger and strength, and therefore refused to find a partner, or if a new child in the group found it difficult to choose a partner. This kind of attitude on the part of the group conductors was a vivid representation of the feelings of mutuality and the capacity for concern as outlined in Winnicott (2012/1984; 2018). In counting, the group conductors employ the fingers of one hand while keeping up with each digit counted, flexing and stretching the forearm. In this way, it is easier to remain at the desired counting speed of ten seconds. In addition, the children who are willing to count have a clear visual representation of the pace. The shouting should be lively in the sense of not holding back any tension or energy (Casriel, 1972), whilst not promoting any dysregulation. Associative thinking was also encouraged between the bataca partners; for instance, after long breaks like holidays, one was able to say: 'I missed you' or 'I hate you although I have missed you'. This can be perceived either as the 'exchange of insults', in Bach and Goldberg's (1976, p. 218) terms, or as offering a neutral space for the expression of aggressive feelings triggered by the separation. In relation to the end-of-fight parting gestures, initially, immediately after the fight, the children were unable to realise that this belonged to the process. The group conductors had to repeatedly remind the participants to use such gestures so that the children could consciously perceive the role of their bataca partner. In this way, anger and physical strength may be experienced and understood as a positive experience. As time went by, the children repeatedly wanted Leticia and Niko to start the bataca fight, the same as the mirror aspect of Gestalt therapy. Watching the eclectic group conductors fight kept them amused. Either at Christmas or the summer farewell, when girls' and boys' groups were put together, it was possible to increase the number of fights and to encourage fights between girls and boys. The idea could be introduced in play as a challenge of courage, or even as a means of assessing the seriousness of the children's desire to play together in a feasible, non-gendered group.

1.2 Primal scream (as a closing ritual)

The primal scream is a simple, shared way of releasing any frustration that may have arisen during the group session (Casriel, 1972). In fact, it is a farewell greeting based on physical expressions (screaming) and hand contact – serving the same purpose as the parting gesture in the bataca fights. All the children stand in a circle holding hands, and on the count of 'one' by the group conductors, the hands are taken up with an inhale and down with an exhale. On the count of 'two', the same procedure is followed, and on the count of 'three', everyone lets out a collective shout on the exhale while holding their hands down and pressing their neighbour's hands together firmly with both hands. The group ends with this.

Guidance notes: After the collective shout, it is recommended that each member of the group shout alone, demonstrating the power of their voice, accompanied by any anger and/or fear. This creates unity or 'shared meaning communication'. To avoid conflicts about who starts or finishes, the eclectic group conductors should stand side-by-side and one of the eclectic group conductors lead the first individual call. The sequence of the next individual shouts continues clockwise until the last shout is led by the other eclectic group conductor.

Sometimes girls and boys do not like to make physical contact. Therefore, the children can be positioned in such a way that the boys and girls stand next to each other. However, to complete a circle, a girl and a boy must hold hands at one point. Religious or cultural reasons may also play a role. There is no perfect solution to this challenge. One can insist that they only hold on to a little finger or at least hold each other's sleeve. In addition, a group leader can ask if one of the children is feeling brave enough to swap places, regardless of whether they are a boy or a girl. Sometimes, other children offer help of their own accord. One should also not push this too much. The important thing is to reinforce the impression of togetherness.

Finally, it is worth highlighting that both the rituals adopted (the bataca fight and the primal scream) intend to trigger the integration of all dimensions of the child, i.e., to encourage the child's senses, body, emotions and mind to work in unity (or in homeostasis).

2 Non-ritualised anger management

2.1 Mashoonga fight

The mashoonga bat is a modern variation of the bo, a traditional Japanese fighting stick. With these slightly elastic sticks, which are covered with shock-absorbing foam, one can do a kind of sword fight. The aim of the game is to touch the opponent with the tip of the mashoonga bat. Apart from having fun and being able to punch and shout, it is all about skill. Longer than the batacas, they are less padded and therefore easier to hold in terms of weight and are more dynamic in terms of movement. They require more refined sensorimotor skills from the children, as in a fight, the children must be able to identify hits well and simultaneously attack and defend themselves. In bataca fights, this type of challenge is lacking, as the focus is simply on the use of one's own potential strength and thus on the recognition of it. The mashoonga fight's rules remain the same: hits to the head and genitals, and to the breast area for girls, are expressly forbidden. If the rules of the game are deliberately broken, the child will be automatically expelled from the group session. The two players touch a spot marked on the floor with the tip of their mashoonga bats. When the tips of their mashoonga bats touch each other, the fight begins. Depending on the group size and the number of planned fights, the number of points at which the fight ends is determined, e.g., whoever reaches three points first. The name 'sword fight' is appropriate to describe a mashoonga fight because with a sword even the smallest blows would result in injury, but for our purposes the blows result in points. This picture is easy to explain to the children. Each child should point out hits to the other, thus creating a 'field of honesty', as it is often difficult to tell from the outside, in the role of referee, whether a hit has been scored or not. One's own honesty is an important aspect of impulse control related to coping with the possible role of winner or loser – a striking difference to bataca fighting.

Guidance notes: The idea is to support the children in practising their concentration, self-control and acknowledgment of hits. The eclectic group conductors must first of all demonstrate the fight in a lively way, for instance by verbally teasing each other. They should also become members of the teams and fight together with the children. In a mixed group, the girls versus boys game mode makes sense since the challenge is not in the strength of the punch, but rather in the skills. Girls are on an equal physical footing in this type of game. The girls sit on one side of the room and the boys on the other side. Once they have finished battling, they are allowed to pass the mashoonga on to a different child. This creates a new pairing. The small and big round mode from the bataca fight may be adopted in this game. The number of points defines the duration of the fight. A small number of points reduces the waiting time of the remaining group. If the atmosphere in the group becomes intense, it is preferable to run several short rounds.

If a conflict arises in the group, particularly with one of the eclectic group conductors, it would be advisable to invite the child involved in the conflict to a 'sword fight' with that conductor. This can release tensions, and the child's anger and aggression can be properly expressed and contained by the eclectic conductor, who should try to put into words the emotions involved in the fight ('maternal reverie' approach).

2.2 Belt-pulling fight

The belt-pulling fight is performed with judo or karate belts. Similar to Bataca, the main challenge here is to use and recognise one's own potential strength, but there is also the idea of being part of a team. A belt-pulling fight consists of a preparatory phase in which two teams are formed and each child creates an imaginary name for him/herself and communicates this to the leaders of the game. The idea is to use physical strength to its maximum potential and to draw strength from the imaginary figure and/or to use this figure to move away from oneself. Their names are written down. Very often, children want to have the same names, for instance, if the name is 'Batman', then this becomes 'Batman 2', 'Batman 3', etc. – this method is welcomed by the children. Then, the group is divided into two teams. Each team moves to opposite sides of the room. In the starting position, one of the hands of each child in the team should be touching the wall. They are also allowed to stretch out their other hand towards the person struggling with the belt. The centre line of the room can be marked with tape to make it clear that all the children should start from the same position. Next, two children are randomly called out by their fantasy name, e.g., 'Batman 2 vs. Batman 3'. This is followed by the second command, 'On your marks, get set, go!' On 'go', one of the eclectic group conductors throws the belt on the floor with each end of the belt pointing to the respective sides of the room. The two named children should then rush off and grab one end of the belt each and drag it with all their strength towards their team. The winner is the player who manages to bring the opponent into his team's field and at the same time touches the free hand of one of his team members, whose other hand is fixed to the wall.

Guidance notes: The rules of the game can be monitored all at once. One of the eclectic group conductors throws the belt on 'go', while the other keeps the score sheet, records which child from which team has won and makes sure that teams do not remove their hands which are touching the wall. By choosing teams, younger and older children should be well mixed in both teams, otherwise unnecessary frustration may be felt by the team members. Releasing the belt when one realises that they have lost is a violation of the rules, as the other person will certainly fall down suddenly and may get hurt – this results in a warning (rule 11, in chapter 5, section 5.3.1.), followed by a deduction in the team's score by one point. The same reduction is applicable if a team member has not kept one hand on the wall. Another variant of the game is when one of the eclectic group conductors joins a team and becomes a member of it, which is more than welcome by the children. In this case, the other group conductor takes full responsibility for leading the game. Finally, a classic game of tug-of-war may take place as a constructive way of re-establishing a sense of unity. Here, both teams compete against each other, including one group conductor in each team.

2.3 Boxing with/without a punching bag

Boxing using a punching bag: for this game, two pairs of boxing gloves in different colours, a bell and a portable punching bag are needed. One of the eclectic group conductors should hang the punching bag over his or her shoulder, whilst the bell should also be held in his or her free hand. For each hit against the punching bag, the group conductor will ring the bell. The loudness and intensity of the bell's ring will provide the boxer with acoustic feedback on his or her boxing strength potential whilst motivating him or her onwards. Each child then, in turn, boxes for ten seconds. Similar to the bataca fight, the eclectic group conductors count vigorously, together with the group, up to ten. Whilst one child is boxing, the next one gets help from the others with putting on the boxing gloves. The game continues, with each child having a go, until everyone has had a turn.

Boxing without a punching bag: for this game, two pairs of boxing gloves in different colours and two head protectors with face shields (available in martial arts stores) are needed, as two children will now box against each other. These head protectors must be designed so that the head can be hit without causing injury because, as in adult boxing, the head is now also a hitting area. No boxing lower than belly button height is allowed. It is recommended that the children perform a few very light and reciprocal blows to their heads to give them an idea of the effect of an impact. Then, the children decide when to start by 'boxing' each other, wearing both boxing gloves. The round lasts ten seconds and the children sitting in a circle may cheer by counting and shouting. If one fighter drops or if they get tangled up the bout is interrupted. If the boxers are unequal in age, weight, size or gender, a handicap may be applied, i.e., only fighting with one arm or fighting whilst kneeling. For young fighters, caution towards oneself and the other fighter can be applied, i.e., 'half strength' can be requested. Making the group circle large to enlarge the arena may also be worthwhile.

Guidance notes: The first manner of boxing involves anger expression combined with caring. The latter can be seen not only among the children when they help each other put on the gloves, but also towards the eclectic group conductor who carries the punching bag. By holding the punching bag, the eclectic group conductor enables the children simultaneously to experience how to manage their expression of anger and/or feelings of frustration (by boxing) linked to concern (not hurting the group conductor) – a similar experience to a historical (archaic) one when the infant was unable to cope with innate aggressive forces linked to the task of living and loving (Winnicott et al., 2012/1984, pp. 71–85; see also Winnicott, 2014). Indeed, our advice is that the female group conductor carries the punching bag. The second manner of boxing, which is more akin to 'adult boxing', obviously attracts more boys than girls, as firstly it is basically a game of strength, and secondly the girls are less familiar with expressing their anger in this manner. Boys should be warned at times not to hit in an uncoordinated manner, using only brute force, but rather to implement mental and motor control. While the girls should preferably be assisted by the female group conductor who offers herself as a fighting partner.

This game (in both forms) should be played towards the end of the consolidation phase, as not only the bonds between the participants will be stronger then, but also anger management has a higher level of representational development.

2.4 Throwing games with a ball

For 'dodgeball' and 'zombie dodgeball', a soft foam ball is needed. The aim of both games is to hit a member of the opposition with the ball anywhere on the body, except the head and genitals. In 'zombie ball', the game starts when one of the group conductors throws the ball into the room. Anyone can grab the ball. A child who grabs the ball is allowed to move a maximum of three steps and must then throw the ball to another person. Should a child be hit by the ball, then that child must quit the game and wait until three more children have been hit. As soon as the fourth child is hit, the first child can return to the game – appropriate training for low frustration tolerance. Should a child catch the ball and not drop it, he/she must shout 'zombie' loudly. In this case, the three previously eliminated players can automatically return to the game, while the player who threw the ball to the 'zombie' is eliminated from the game. In 'burn ball', the playing field is divided into two halves, in which each team is positioned. Each half is in turn divided into two parts: the playing field and, at its back, the graveyard for the opposing team as illustrated in Figure 7.1.

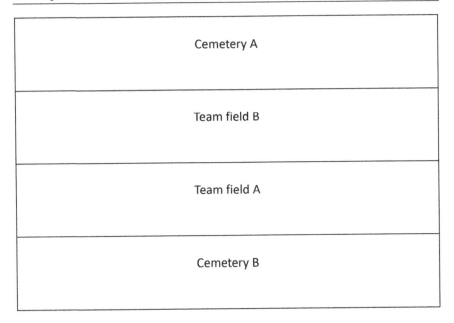

Figure 7.1 Playing court.

Should a member of team A be hit, he or she must move to graveyard A and from there, he or she can hit team B members with the ball but cannot return to team A's field. Should there be no hit, it is the turn of the team that grabs the ball in their respective playing field. The winner is the team that successfully moves all members of the opposite team to the graveyard.

Guidance notes: The 'zombie dodgeball' variant is an impulsive and non-team game that trains individual spatial awareness combined with preventive perception while strengthening frustration tolerance levels. 'Dodgeball', on the other hand, involves an active cooperative playing function. The group conductors should select the variant that is more suited to the level of frustration management in the group or more suited to the group's needs. However, both should be adopted from the middle of the consolidation phase onwards and they are also intended for large groups (N ≥ 8).

2.5 Water fight

There are two versions of the game 'water fight'. For the first one, the group is divided into two teams. Each player gets a disposable cup and clamps it in their mouth. Then, they have to run, one after the other, to the washing tub, fill the cup with water there, run back again with the cup in their mouth, high-five the next child and pour the water into the team bucket. The team that fills the team bucket first or has more water in it after a certain time wins.

For the second version of the game, a large number of balloons are filled with water and distributed in washtubs on the lawn. Everyone takes as many water balloons as possible and hits each other with them. There are no explicit rules, except no hitting the face or the genitals, as well as being careful not to throw the balloons too hard.

Guidance notes: Children have a lot of fun with both versions of 'water fight'; however, the most fun to be had is when they can get the eclectic group conductors wet. A water fight is a useful game (especially if adopted in the last group meeting before the summer break) for processing frustrations and the mourning triggered by the upcoming separation phase, in a fun and constructive way.

2.6 Haka

The Maori dance Haka means 'dance' or 'song with dance' and is a symbolic martial dance without weapons for motivating oneself and intimidating the opponents. We took up this basic idea and turned it into a game. Two teams are formed: mostly, the girls position themselves behind the female group conductor and the boys behind the male one, facing each other head-on. Alongside this, a Haka melody with loud shouting and jeering is played on the music box. The children are tasked with imitating the game leader in front of them and looking at the other group, beating their chests, stomping hard on the ground, yelling together with words like 'Huga', 'Eia' or similar, sticking out their tongues and grimacing. The children get involved with the energy of the Haka.

Guidance notes: This is a game that involves the five basic channels of human perception according to Gestalt therapy. To move into expressive dance movements, it is advised that the music is listened to beforehand, that the group conductors are observe and that the basic movements are practised. Performing must be done with great confidence to engage the children in the dance, as well as for anger and rage to be expressed.

3 Ego-strengthening: Promotion of social togetherness

3.1 Card game

Everyone sits in a circle of chairs. A deck of German playing cards made up of four symbols are used, namely acorns, hearts, leaves and bells. These symbols are introduced so that they are understood by everyone. Everyone gets a playing card and keeps it in their hand, noting the symbol and the chair they are sitting on. Then, the cards are given back. Now, the game leader reveals one card after the other and names the symbol on the card. All the children with the corresponding symbol may move one seat to the right. If someone is sitting there, they have to sit on their lap. If several people are sitting on top of each other, only the top child may move to the right; the others are blocked, even if their symbol is drawn. When everyone has moved, the next card is turned over. The winner is the first person to sit back on their starting chair.

Guidance notes: This card game is basically a game of chance, as its outcome is not influenced by mental or physical abilities. However, it has a cathartic character, as it often leads to situations in which there is prolonged and strong physical contact. In this blockade, each player has to work out his own frustration, in a fun and familiar way. On a symbolic level, it is an approach that allows us to process feelings of powerlessness in the face of reality. No wonder this has been one of the children's favourite games in all the groups and they very much respected the outcome of the game. We never had any difficulties with the game itself being questioned, but there were many attempts at cheating (e.g., moving one seat further than allowed) that were discussed and resolved in the group. This helped us a lot with relationship building. As a deciding game (see chapter 6), the winner, who has to choose the next game, often encounters pressure from their peers to fulfil their wishes – a fruitful moment for strengthening resilience. However, if the situation escalates, then one of the group conductors should take the winner outside of the room, so that he or she can freely decide by him or herself which game will be played. Individual tasks can be given to children in the course of the game, e.g., distributing and collecting the cards at the beginning. If one or more children refuse to sit on the lap of a child of the opposite sex, it is important to build bridges. First of all, one should emphasise the nature of the game and ask them to join in, because others also 'dare' to do this. However, if this does not work, an object, e.g., a pen, can be offered. This should be held by both to show their attachment. It is not recommended to propose that they just stand in front of the other person without sitting down, as the feeling of being blocked out, without physical contact, increases the temptation to cheat and just keep moving. Persistent cheating can lead to a restart of the game if the cheating means that the positive atmosphere in the group is threatened. In this case, clear intervention is needed towards the cheating child. An additional motivating factor for winning is the incentive of being able to decide on the next game at the end. In any case, the children enjoyed sitting on the laps of the eclectic group conductors and vice versa.

Even though this is a well-known game and is played by two adults, depending on the characteristics of the institution (e.g., religious) in which the group meets, it is recommended to ask for parental permission to play it. In this way, any kind of misunderstanding regarding the act of sitting on the lap (a physical contact) can be avoided. Alternatively, as stated above, instead of sitting on the lap, 'sticks' could be used (so that each player has to hold one end of the stick as a symbol of connection). It is up to the eclectic group conductors to find the appropriate solution.

3.2 Being glued to the wall

The primary goals of this game are the promotion of trust, responsibility and cooperation (Häfele, 2009 p. 38). A child chooses to be glued to the wall of his or her own free will. In general, it was the person who won the card game. 'Being glued to the wall' consists of a child wearing a protective helmet, standing on a chair with his or her back against the wall (see Figure 5.3 in chapter 5), while the group's task is to tape this child to the wall in such a way that he or she is only held in place by tape so that the chair can then be removed. The task of the group conductors is to monitor and support the work of the group and the child being taped, while dealing with possible conflicts arising from the situation (see guidance notes). The tape should not be passed over the neck, as the child will slide down a few centimetres when the chair is pulled and he or she will hang free for a moment. Tape pressing against the throat should be avoided. One of the group conductors, or a reliable child, will, after consultation, slowly pull the chair away. While doing so, the child taped to the wall receives clear eye contact so that he or she feels confident and 'held up'. It is recommended that this tense moment is supported with words, such as: *'Are you scared? I would be too! But you don't have to be – I'm with you!'* For the children who are glued, it is a unique experience. Taking a group photo of this unusual situation and keeping it for the photo album to be given to the group at the farewell group meeting is a good idea.

Guidance notes: 'Being glued to the wall' is a team exercise for building trust and sometimes requires a high level of rule-making because the person who is glued to the wall entrusts himself or herself in a defenceless position, which the group conductors have to protect them. The unfamiliar setting opens up new spaces of experience, and the verbalisation of the experience comes into its own. In this way, the latent fields of conflict, such as power-lessness, fear, mutual prejudice, attempts at mutual humiliation, mechanisms of exclusion and feelings such as mistrust may be addressed gradually. Check the wall beforehand to make sure that adhesive tape will stick well and reserve this wall as the place for this game, as the wall paint will certainly be damaged by the adhesive tape. However, the wall can be restored if one combines it, for example, with a painting project (see description below). For this game, a small group size of up to eight children is recommended ($N \leq 8$).

3.3 Rubber chicken

The aim of the game is that all the children steal the rubber chicken from the group conductor when he/she is not looking, and then everyone returns together to the starting point without him/her knowing who has the rubber chicken – this requires coordinated teamwork. At the beginning, until the game is understood by everyone, one of the group conductors should join the team. Before the game starts, the children and the other group conductor line up on opposite walls of a large room, as shown in Figure 7.2. In the children's play area, a line is marked on the floor behind which all the children should stay until the game starts and after it ends.

The rubber chicken is placed on the floor in front of the one of the group conductors. The game starts when he or she turns around and says, 'Yes, where on earth is my rubber chicken?' By turning his or her back to the children, the conductor can no longer see them – the perfect time for the children to move towards the rubber chicken. In this way, the children also have an acoustic clue for recognising when they can be seen and when they cannot. As soon as they are visible to the group conductor again, they remain frozen. If another child moves, the whole group has to start again. As soon as the rubber chicken is no longer in its place, i.e., it has been 'stolen', the group conductor, after completing a 360 degree turn, is allowed to guess who is holding the chicken. If the conductor guesses incorrectly, the child accused of having the object stretches out his/her arms and the game continues. If the group leader has guessed correctly, the whole group has to start again. The rubber chicken was originally a dog toy for playing fetch and also squeaks when pressed because it has a built-in whistle. Of course, it could be any soft toy, but it is the squeaking that makes the chicken very appealing to the

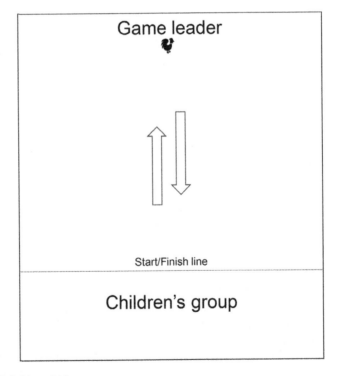

Figure 7.2 Rubber chicken.

children. In addition, they have to be very careful when holding the chicken so that the group conductor cannot identify who is holding it. The rubber chicken should not be held by only one child. It must be passed to another child without being thrown. If the group is large enough, two teams can be formed, e.g., girls vs. boys. In this case, the eclectic group conductors join a team (a second rubber chicken is needed) and he or she takes on the role of 'mum/dad', encouraging the children to work together as a team (family) and making sure that no rules are broken. The victory point is awarded to the team (or family) that crosses their initial marked line first, with all its members and, of course, has also 'stolen' the rubber chicken and brought it back to their territory.

Guidance notes: This game is perfect for adequately and effectively addressing antisocial topics, as it provides multiple opportunities for challenging 'ego-relatedness' via several real situations, such as the act of taking something, the feeling of being watched and controlled by 'mum and dad', the prospect of being caught and held responsible for something and all this happening together with other children. Even if the aim of the game is not achieved, the children have a lot of fun in between, which contributes to the development of the relationship between the children and the eclectic group conductors. The game requires coordination and teamwork skills, combined with trust and patience. Once everyone is familiar with the game, the eclectic group conductors can increase the emotional tension by making the rubber chicken a transitional object and building a relationship with it while the children are in the frozen position. This way, the rubber chicken can be 'flirted' with, picked up and comforted like a baby, talked to or even taken to the toilet – one's imagination is allowed to run wild. In this way, the children are challenged to remain immobile, even when they want to laugh or express their own impatience. What is crucial is the flexibility and spontaneity of the eclectic group conductors in meeting the appropriate level of challenge depending on the matrix of the group's dynamic.

3.4 Musical chairs

Chairs are set up (there is always one less chair than the total number of people present) in a circle. Players must move around the chairs while the music is playing, but when it stops, they have to sit down on a chair. Whoever ends up without a chair to sit on at the end loses that round. The game is played until one player is left.

Guidance notes: The group conductors should divide their tasks: one of them plays along with the children, the other controls the music. This is basically a coordination game, yet the group conductors may introduce relational experiences, for instance should children get knocked out, they may either sit outside the circle and help the conductor to control the music (this also applies to a child who does not want to play along) or they may even 'dance along' with the group conductor on the side-lines. The latter in particular is recommended as it shows the child is still having fun despite 'being a loser'. There may be situations where one child sits on another, e.g., on his or her lap. In this case, the group conductors have to intervene and highlight the fact this isn't allowed to happen in order to promote understanding.

3.5 Musical statues

One person controls the music. When the music plays, everyone moves and dances. When the music stops, the children freeze in their last position until the music starts up again. The last person to move is eliminated. The game continues until only one child remains.

Guidance notes: This game involves the five basic channels of human perception according to Gestalt therapy (Oaklander, 1988): movement, auditory processing and responding, attention and control, and balance. It is advisable to let a child choose the music so that it matches the general taste in music of the group, making as many children feel as included as possible. One of the group conductors, together with a child, determines who was the last to move in their opinion. If there is any confusion, the children can start dancing again without anyone getting eliminating. It may be that the children do not want to stop dancing, but rather want to show each other dancing movements, following each other's movements, dancing in time with each other, doing a circle dance or a polonaise, etc. In contrast to musical chairs, musical statues is less competitive; it leads to more interaction, particularly with regards to creative expressions of body language. As in musical chairs, the children who are eliminated can help the conductor to control the music.

3.6 Blind cow

For this game, one of the group conductors is blindfolded and tries to catch the children. Each child that is caught is then blindfolded and helps the group conductor to catch the others. The winner is the child without a blindfold at the end.

Guidance notes: This game is perfect for successfully addressing polarities, as it involves a shift in the children's roles from 'repelling the group conductor' to ' being by his or her side and supporting him or her' – two quite opposing situations, which in the game may be experienced as integrative, given that all the children remain in the game.

3.7 Carrot pulling

The children form a circle (with or without the eclectic group conductors – it is up to the children), lie on their stomachs on the floor with their heads towards the centre of the circle and link their hands and arms like a chain: they are the carrots rooted in the ground. Shoes must be taken off. A child, alone or with a group conductor, or even just the group conductor(s), is (are) the farmer and will attempt to 'harvest' a carrot by pulling hard on the legs until a child can no longer hold on to the other children. This might only work after several attempts, as the children lying on the ground aim to hold on to each other. As soon as a carrot is harvested, that child will help the farmer to keep on pulling the other carrots. The process goes on like this until the last two carrots have been pulled. Children are not allowed to pull the legs up and just let them fall, as this may hurt.

Guidance notes: This game highlights the importance of cohesion within a group and thus the feeling of belonging, which is essential for a child's identity. If the group is united and everyone is linking onto each other like a chain, it is extremely difficult for an outsider to act against this group. It is certainly a game that releases a lot of physical energy from all the members of the group at the same time. Aggressive energy is processed together in the group – a sense of unity. Similar to the game 'blind cow', the children change roles during the game to achieve opposing goals. Depending on the ground conditions, it may be useful to wear long sleeves to avoid abrasions. Covering the ground with a large sheet is another immediate solution. According to the age and size of the children, the game may start with two children being the farmers.

4 Ego-strengthening: Family-like experiences

4.1 Singing

Singing a song in a chaotic situation helps calm the group down. Firstly, the singer – in this instance, one of the eclectic group conductors – should definitely be feeling calm in order to start singing. The singer's sense of security will automatically be reflected in the group's dynamics, as he/she starts to distance him/herself from the chaos, while giving the group this sense of security – a new symbolic shape. Any song can be chosen – it simply needs to be filled with emotion on the part of the singer. If the children are not familiar with it, either with the melody or the language, all the better.

Guidance notes: This approach is associated with what Bion (1984a; 1984b) referred to as 'maternal reverie' and 'container-contained interaction' – a situation similar to early childhood moments when the mother's voice has a calming effect on the infant. By introducing a melody in a chaotic group situation, children can get in touch with their past (archaic) experiences when as infants they were at the mercy of inner chaos and were held by someone (usually the mother).

4.2 Dancing

Dancing was incorporated in various forms into the group activities, along with the above-mentioned games. For instance, after a team had won a game, sometimes this led to spontaneous polonaises including all the children. The song 'I feel good' by James Brown was adapted to a 'winner's ritual' with the following lyrical variation, *'I feel good – ba da da, ba da da, I have won, ba da da, ba da da, so nice, so nice, I feel good, good, good!'* In this amusing setting, it was easier to deal with the 'losers' disappointment, since there was no pejorative, but rather an expression of a good mood. Another variation is for the girls to dance the way the boys typically dance or the other way around, which was often very funny for everyone, especially when the boys showed off cool dance moves. Occasionally, the eclectic group conductors danced a salsa for the group's opening whilst the children came into the room and took their seats. The eclectic group conductors may perform any dance. What is most important is that they should dance together as a couple. This variation creates a peaceful setting for the beginning of a group session, similar to 'Mum and Dad' being in a good relationship, as well as having some of their own fun.

Guidance notes: Dancing is adopted as a means of communication for bringing ambiguities together. As for the last variation, it may happen that a few children try to interrupt the dance and get in the middle of the couple to separate them. In such cases, the group conductors should continue dancing (not allowing the separation), but then put into words the child's expression of aggressive energy. In this way, 'ego-connectedness' issues are properly dealt with.

4.3 Cooking

Cooking is a common activity at the end-of-term parties before the holidays or other breaks in winter. Generally, the group is divided into a small group of up to three children during the 'welcome timeslot'. Each group is in the kitchen with one of the group conductors while the others do a play activity with the other group conductor in the nearby room. The groups then switch. For instance, during pizza-making, there were times when the teams had a competition for which team could make the tastiest pizza.

Guidance notes: When cooking, the children carried out new duties, such as taking out the rubbish, cleaning up, setting the table and preparing food. In short, this enabled the children to experience intimate domestic situations which are ordinarily associated with family-of-origin situations.

4.4 Physical exercises

In the group formation phase, the children were interested in encountering each other through joint physical exercises, like arm presses/push-ups or gymnastics/yoga. The goal was to show each other how strong or how limber they are, or how well they can keep their balance. They were also excited to find out the sporty skills that the female and male conductors were able to perform.

Guidance notes: It is important that both group conductors come up with ideas for physical exercises and challenge each other in a friendly way during the game. In addition, the group conductors should draw attention to the diversity of their bodies – basic training for the practical formation of an understanding of diversity.

4.5 Celebrating birthdays

The 'farewell timeslot' of the last group meeting of the month was partially reserved for celebrating that month's birthdays. A cake was baked by the group conductor herself, and preparing the birthday table was designed to be a group task – a familiar setting with lively conversation. As mentioned in chapter 6, celebrating a birthday involves bringing the groups of girls and boys together for a short period of time. It is also a suitable approach for sensitising both groups to future collective activities, such as the ones that will take place before Christmas and the summer holidays – a barometer for assessing the group's maturity.

Guidance notes: Celebrating birthdays should not be seen as a ritual, as it makes no sense to share a birthday cake if the group is engaged in serious antisocial behaviour during the meeting. Such a cake would be a reward for rule-breaking behaviour. If a birthday party were to be cancelled because of antisocial behaviour, an arrangement could be made for the birthday child (ren) of that month to use the disappointing behaviour as an opportunity for reflection. In such cases, provided the special agreement has been honoured, the birthday child(ren) will be rewarded with a special little extra cake the following month. It is important to make this clear to the children so that they understand the meaning of the celebration.

4.6 Painting project

The painting project is an activity to be adopted at the end of the consolidation phase onwards, after the relationships with the eclectic group conductors are well-established. This activity was conceived as a way of strengthening the children's roles towards society, as well as a means of assessing the children's performance during an entire Saturday session together, with the eclectic group conductors. The idea is to paint either the communal walls of the shared housing for refugees that were marked with some graffiti and sexual symbols, or the wall badly damaged by the game 'being glued to the wall'. The group of children should not be larger than 12 participants, who should be divided into two sub-groups that will rotate. Each group conductor is responsible for one sub-group. While one sub-group paints a piece of the damaged wall, the other sub-group paints T-shirts in the group room. These T-shirts are intended to be worn on a group excursion at a later date – a transient object between the two activities that creates the sense of forward planning, coupled with the meaning behind cause and effect.

Guidance notes: Being together intensively for a day encourages many family-like processes, such as on a communication level 'Look what I have made!' … 'Yes, that looks great!' … 'I need your help!' … 'Yes, I'll be right there!' Or even with regards to actions: occasions for chatting, drinking and eating together. Undeniably, unexpected situations, i.e., conflict among the children, may also arise and then a communal search for solutions is called for.

4.7 Excursion

As previously mentioned, the excursion is linked to the outcome of the painting project and may therefore be perceived as a reward for it. This means that for the excursion activity, unusually, the group becomes a closed group – strictly restricted to the participants of the painting project.

Guidance notes: The nature and location of the excursion should be discussed together in the group. For example, if it is in the summer and the children would like to go to the swimming pool, make sure they can all swim. Otherwise, get together in search of solutions. Written parental consent is also needed and, depending on the group size, some of the parents may be required to participate.

4.8 Film evening

The film evening takes place during a normal group meeting. If the film is longer than 90 minutes, then it should be spread over two meetings so that there was enough time for arrivals, and breaks for popcorn, cola and going to the toilet, as well as for cleaning-up and for proper farewells. Seats for the eclectic group conductors are labelled in advance with a name tag and are situated in the middle. Children sit around them in order to emphasise the fact that it is a film evening with the eclectic group conductors. Afterwards, cleaning up and sweeping the room together form part of the film evening.

Guidance notes: A film evening should be carried out from the farewell phase onwards, as the primary aim is to build a family atmosphere whilst deepening the bond amongst the group. This can be achieved by simple means, such as eating popcorn together, tidying up the room together, chatting and sharing 'oohs' and 'ahhs' during the film screening. At this stage, the achievement of the 'shared meaning communication' is quite clear; otherwise, the group would be unable to enjoy watching a film in German together, considering all the cultural differences among the children and the eclectic group conductors. For all the children, it is certainly a new family-like experience when compared to watching a film in their own family circle in their respective mother tongues.

4.9 Photo project

From the start of the farewell phase, at every group meeting, a timeline photo gallery is set up in the group room before the children arrive. Once the doors of the group room are opened 15 minutes before its start, the children can admire their photos.

Guidance notes: This very simple project is of great value as it helps the children to recover their sense of time continuity, as well as triggering an awareness of their own timeline (Castrechini-Franieck, 2022). In the case of refugee children, the latter has mostly been lost by many of them, due to their families fleeing from their homeland, and continuity has become a longed-for need.

5 Ego-strengthening: Encouraging the imagination

5.1 Dream bag

This is a large suitcase containing old skirts, dresses, shoes (including high heels for women), wigs, glasses, caps, belts, football shirts, blouses/shirts and pullovers. One may play with it in two different ways. 1) Everyone is allowed to choose something, dress up themselves and introduce themselves afterwards as a character. For example, on one occasion, a video was recorded and it was very funny and entertaining to watch the children perform in the video clip afterwards. The video was watched several times by the group. 2) The eclectic group conductors were dressed up by the group. Once, the group made a mockery of Niko because he was very late for the group. For not respecting one of the 14 rules of the group (be on time), he had to dress up as a woman as a sanction. The clothes he had to wear were decided by the group in advance before he arrived, as reported in Castrechini-Franieck and Bittner (2022b, pp. 177–180). On another occasion, Leticia was supposed to dress up like a man and Niko like a woman.

Guideline notes: This game is best suited to an advanced stage of the group with a greater degree of familiarity, as its focus is mainly on placing oneself in the role of the opposite gender in a playful and fun way, for which there are rarely opportunities in everyday life. The introduction of gender role swapping should be a task performed by the eclectic group conductors themselves. Consequently, many children will find new experiences for themselves in a flexible way, free from role allocations. In simpler terms, they can freely practice 'shared meaning communication' in a playful way.

5.2 'Excrement machine' or simply 'poo machine' (to mimic the children's language)

This requires brown modelling clay (good for shaping piles of poo) and modelling clay figure sets with which one can create one's own poo monsters with funny eyes, arms, noses and other accessories. One can also replace the brown modelling clay with a mixture of chocolate-hazelnut cream and flour. Many thoughts about how to deal with their own 'poo' are triggered for the children by the 'making process', which thus leads to very frank conversations. With the older children going through puberty, this game then led to the creation of penises and vaginas and an interchange of questions around sexuality.

Guidance notes: This method is best suited to an advanced stage of the group where there is a higher level of familiarity, as a playful openness is required for the process of sharing intimate matters. The aim of this game is to provide a neutral and transitional space in which 'taboo' issues can be dealt with in an open and non-moral context – therefore, the practice of 'shared meaning communication' must be carried out by the group conductors. For example, once when the eclectic group conductors were asked how often they 'poop' during the day, the children got their answer in a respectful manner. Or, taking the case of modelling penises and vaginas using playdough, from our perspective, this is a more refined way for the expression of sexuality (within the group), rather than them being scribbled (secretly) on the communal walls of the shared housing for refugees.

6 Reflection

Reflection aims to encourage feelings to be expressed as well as to put them into words, thus improving the ability to communicate (Bion, 1984a; 1984b).

6.1 Transcriptions

As explained in chapters 5 and 6, written transcription belongs to one of the four basic procedures adopted by the eclectic group conductors outside the group setting.

Guidance notes: It is an attempt to practise the maternal reverie (Bion, 1984a; 1984b). This manner of reflection contributed to a significant improvement in our work with the children, as their needs could be better understood.

6.2 Thumbprint

As outlined in chapter 6, this is a communal reflection with the children that belongs to the farewell timeslot.

Guidance notes: At the beginning, during the group formation phase, children make use of this reflection time both to complain about minor moments of silliness (in order to get more attention) and to throw chairs on the floor (to show their anger) at the end of the reflection time. These behaviour patterns seem more like a kind of resistance to the feelings of separation, because towards the middle of the consolidation phase, children start to share their ideas and/or wishes for the next group meetings. New ideas for a game and/or for an excursion and/or for a movie night should be reflected upon as a group, in accordance with the second T-WAS main tenet, as described earlier in chapter 6.

7 Contact design during the COVID-19

In March 2020, when the COVID-19 pandemic started, we had just finished our first group session (T), which lasted two years. Our second group (S) was due to finish in July and an initial session with a new group (our third group) (B) had just started (see details in chapter 8). The unforeseen lockdown caused everything to come to an abrupt standstill. Then, in May, new-found contact with the children started in connection with a new concept for group work based on a sequence of letters, phone calls and self-produced mini-movies with the eclectic group conductors as the protagonists. On a weekly basis, we phoned the children at the times when 'normally' group appointments would have taken place and we also sent two letters, which were kindly delivered by the social workers at the shared housing for refugees. One letter was planned to reach the children the day before the phone call; the other letter, the day after. The content of the first letter was concerned with our wish to call them, whilst the content of the second letter referred to the feedback about our call and also to the announcement of the next short film (an example of both letters can be found in Appendix 7.1). Immediately after the phone calls, a short film was sent to the children via WhatsApp. In order to be allowed to use WhatsApp, we had obtained the consent forms from the children's parents. The topics of the films were intended to maintain light-hearted contact and to make the children smile. For instance, the children were able to watch Niko and Leticia growing up from toddlers to the adults they are today. In other films, we cooked our favourite foods. Other times, we set the children riddles and the children could win a prize, like in a raffle, for solving them. Sometimes, we played funny games or even danced or sang together. This was not about our dancing or singing skills but about creating a transitional space in our communication with the children. Then, for two months, in September and October, it was possible to meet again in the S and B shelters of the shared housing for refugees. Since the meeting space in the group rooms was limited, we met outside at a nearby park. Despite the uncomfortable autumn weather and the growing darkness, almost all the children who had been with us before came. In order to keep our distance, the 'bataca fight' was replaced by the 'mashoonga fight' as a starting ritual. Moreover, more throwing games with balls were adopted, as a way of avoiding physical contact. The final ritual, the primal scream, was also run without any hand-holding. From November until mid-December, lockdown restrictions were in place again and we returned to phone calls, letters and films as a way of keeping in touch. The groups ended before the second hard lockdown in December 2020. Shortly before that, we still had the opportunity to say one-to-one farewells with the children in group B and group S as will be described in chapter 8.

In Appendix 7.2, Table 7.1 contains a summary of each self-produced mini-movie, including their respective QR codes and YouTube links. The films have been listed in the table chronologically, according to when they were created, together with information on which group they were produced for. A total of 19 video clips were produced – four of them exclusively for the children in group S (in the farewell phase) and three of them exclusively for the children in group B (in the formation phase). The remaining 12 films were created for both groups. The 20th film in the table with the title 'The Lockdowns' highlights the development of contact building with the children during the lockdowns caused by the COVID-19 pandemic.

(Further details on T-WAS during the COVID-19 pandemic are given in Castrechini-Franieck and Bittner, 2022a, pp. 190–194 and p. 196.)

8 Some personal observations

Practically, we suggest that future eclectic group conductors carry a suitcase with some tools, for example: judo/karate belts, soft balls to play, boxing gloves, music box, card game, 'sticks', protective helmet, tape, rubber chicken, chalk, small bell, etc. All tools must be available, as it is up to the children to decide which game to play at each group meeting. The batakas, mashoongas and pulling sack must be an extra pack. As an approach to anger management in situations of conflict between group members (including conflict with group leaders), non-ritualised anger management games can also be used. In this case, the game should be introduced after an attempt has been made to establish a dialogue between the conflicting members, and should involve verbalising the emotions to enable them to be properly identified and portrayed.

About the creative game itself, most of the games in this chapter are familiar, not new. What makes them creative is the way in which they were interpreted and played by the eclectic group conductors. Starting from their theoretical perspectives, both leaders were able to integrate the concepts of Gestalt therapy into each game (in relation to the expression of aggressive energy via a homeostasis process), together with communication by ontological psychoanalysis (the need for creating a neutral space in which communication can be developed through the container-contained interaction). The variations of the games and their guidance notes are outcomes of this integration. All games can be used as a means of communication. However, the way in which they are played should provide a framework of ego-relatedness for vulnerable children, otherwise the core aim of T-WAS will not be achieved.

Appendix 7.1

Letters to the children:

Hello dear children!   Monday, 22 June 2020

We are sad.

Few of you have returned the consent.

Leticia is crying! She thinks that no one likes her.

I, Niko, try to comfort her, but she doesn't want to be comforted.

She only wants to talk to you.

Please help me! We need more consents!

But we will still send a film out tomorrow.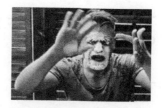
We've put a lot of effort into it. And I, Niko,
got quite a bit...

Take care!

Just in case: Leticia's phone number is **0176–18107150**.

Leticia and Niko
 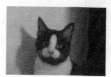

Hello dear children!   Wednesday, 24 June 2020

Yesterday, we talked to many of you.

I, Niko, thank you all! Finally, Leticia is not crying anymore.

This week we got the news that we will not be able to come to your shelter until after the summer holidays.

So, after the summer holidays, the children's group will start again.

Yoo-hoo!   We are very happy!

We will continue to send you new funny films.
Yesterday, we sent a funny film of ours...
Please send us your feedback on yesterday's film!

Those who have not yet given their number (or mum's or dad's), please do so!

Take care!

Just in case: Leticia's phone number is **0176–18107150**.

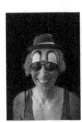   Leticia and Niko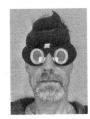

Appendix 7.2

Table 7.1 Short films produced during the COVID-19 pandemic (first and second waves)

Short film	Plot summary	YouTube link
1. 'Fitness in the Forest' (Group S)	In this amateur video, both group conductors, Leticia and Niko, demonstrate several physical workout exercises in the forest, which the children could try out in the park near their camps.	https://youtu.be/5Xr6HeIq62s
2. 'Leticia and Niko Growing-Up' (Groups S and B)	During the first corona wave, the group conductors, Leticia and Niko, start producing the first amateur video for the children. It shows portraits of them in chronological order of their growing up and thus creates a small visual biography. A charming video that won the hearts of the children.	https://youtu.be/VWiKplw78oE
3. 'Leticia and Niko Face-morphing' (Groups S and B)	The group conductors, Leticia and Niko, playfully morph their faces in a second amateur video. An odd video.	https://youtu.be/UZ1LssoiiRw
4. 'Niko Dunked' (Group S)	This amateur video answers questions about Niko, one of the group conductors. After the children had received these questions in the form of a letter a week earlier, Leticia, the other group conductor, now gives the answers in a funny way… it gets a bit dirty on Niko's face.	https://youtu.be/iLvRKYY2O8s
5. 'Niko's Cooking Tip' (Group S)	In this amateur video, one of the group conductors, Niko, introduces one of his favourite dishes – a typical Austrian dish called 'Kaiserschmarrn' (a sweet, sliced pancake with sultanas). He teaches the children step-by-step how to prepare it.	https://youtu.be/AtDJbYv-5e4

Short film	Plot summary	YouTube link
6. 'Leticia's Cooking Tip' (Group S)	In this amateur video, one of the group conductors, Leticia, reveals the secrets of her chocolate cake, which she has often baked for the children's birthdays. In a playful way, she teaches the children how to bake their favourite cake themselves.	https://youtu.be/_hXxK0xyzWk
7. 'Leticia Dunked' (Groups S and B)	Niko, one of the group conductors, answers in a funny way the questions about Leticia, the other group conductor. These questions had been sent to the children by letter a week before. Leticia gets a bit dirty in the face. This time there is a reward for those who have answered the most questions correctly.	https://youtu.be/1mvm-QyhH48
8. 'Leticia's Questions' (Group B)	This amateur video shows the group conductor, Leticia, asking the children questions about herself, which they are asked to answer by indicating true or false. In this initial phase, we had hardly had any contact with the children in this new group and were keen to get to know them.	https://youtu.be/Br6CSF_hHTA
9. 'Niko's Questions' (Group B)	This amateur video shows the group conductor, Niko, asking the children questions about himself, which they are asked to answer by indicating true or false. In this initial phase, we had hardly had any contact with the children in this new group and were keen to get to know them.	https://youtu.be/a0qxw8SecIU
10. 'Leticia and Niko Dunked' (Group B)	This amateur video is a sequel to the 'Leticia's and Niko's Questions' films and answers the questions about the two group conductors, Leticia and Niko. The questions are part of a competition and were sent to the children a week earlier in two separate amateur videos (in each video a group conductor asked questions about themselves). Now each group conductor gives the answers to the questions about the other group conductor, in a very amusing way... it gets a bit dirty on the faces of Leticia and Niko.	https://youtu.be/g9hBdWauqT8

Short film	Plot summary	YouTube link
11. 'Favourite Statue' (Groups S and B)	This amateur video shows three sculptures from the plastic artist Goertz. One week earlier, the children got a letter asking not only for their impressions of the sculptures, but also requesting they choose and give a name to their favourite one.	This short film is not available on YouTube, due to copyright issues
12. 'Guessing Guitar Songs' (Groups S and B)	This amateur video resolves a song guessing game. The children had been asked by letter a week earlier to put the titles of six songs in the right order. The two group conductors played the songs without subtitles (i.e., without a solution), Niko on the guitar and Leticia singing. This video now shows the solution, namely with subtitles. The two group conductors behave comically and sing out of tune.	https://youtu.be/QI_nqncaKis
13. 'Water Fight' (Groups S and B)	This amateur video shows the group conductors, Leticia and Niko, having a water fight on a playground. The water fight was the traditional farewell game for the group before the summer holidays. The aim of this video was to remind the children of this ritual.	https://youtu.be/UDcf0NB4re4
14. 'Have a Great Summer Holidays (2020)' (Groups S and B)	This is the last amateur video before the summer holidays in 2020. The two group conductors, Leticia and Niko, bid the children a warm and playful farewell into the summer holidays. They assure them that they will continue to be there for them after the holidays, even if it is not clear whether this will be in person or in the form of weekly calls, letters and videos.	https://youtu.be/bCrJXSnvCDI
15. 'Switched Voices Joke' (Groups S and B)	The first amateur video produced after two months of face-to-face group meetings in autumn 2020. Each group conductor, Leticia and Niko, tells a joke, although their voices were switched. The aim of this video was to make the children laugh, even though we could no longer meet due to the new second-wave corona restrictions.	https://youtu.be/lUrzfr7m9Lk

Short film	Plot summary	YouTube link
16. 'Clown and Witch' (Groups S and B)	This silent amateur video was produced for Halloween. It tells the story of the witch (Leticia, the group conductor) who tries to trick the clown (Niko, the other group conductor). The poor clown has no chance and ends up in the poop.	https://youtu.be/TTGerP245dI
17. 'Jerusalema' (Groups S and B)	This is an amateur dance video produced to create a guessing game. A week before, the children had received a letter with the following questions: 1) what is the name of the dance? and 2) what did Leticia and Niko eat during it? The winner(s) would be rewarded with a pop-socket, and the children put in a lot of effort.	Due to copyright issues, the music had to be removed from the video. https://youtu.be/a21DVUipy5U
18. 'Sports at Home' (Groups S and B)	In this amateur video, both group conductors, Leticia and Niko, show several amusing sports that the children could try to do at home during lockdown, either with their parents or siblings.	https://youtu.be/UcZtJVRCkQQ
19. 'Cake Fight' (Groups S and B)	This is the last amateur video produced before the end of the groups. In this video, the group conductors, Leticia and Niko, perform an amusing and classic cake fight. The children were delighted with this video, which made it one of their favourite ones.	https://youtu.be/AUwgckB0F14
20. 'The Lockdowns'	From weekly phone calls and letters, to the production of weekly amateur short films, this video is about the author's struggle to keep one children's group alive and the difficulties they had in building a new one – all of this set in the context of the first and second coronavirus waves.	https://youtu.be/7EXt6MQG2iw

Source: From Appendix 9.1, pp. 198–202, *Communicating with Vulnerable Patients: A Novel Psychological Approach*, by Maria Leticia Castrechini Fernandes Franieck, © 2023 Imprint. Published by Routledge, with permission from Taylor and Francis Group.

References

Bach, G.R., and Goldberg, H., 1976. *Creative Aggression*. London: Coventure.

Bion, W.R., 1984a. *Learning from Experience*. London: Maresfield.

Bion, W.R., 1984b. *Second Thoughts: Selected Papers on Psychoanalysis*. London: Routledge.

Blom, R., 2006. *The Handbook of Gestalt Play Therapy: Practical Guidelines for Child Therapists*. London: Jessica Kingsley Publishers.

Casriel, D., 1972. *A Scream Away from Happiness*. New York: Grosset & Dunlap.

Castrechini-Franieck, L., ed., 2022. *Communication with Vulnerable Patients: A Novel Psychological Approach*. London: Routledge.

Castrechini-Franieck, L., and Bittner, N., 2022a. TICA in the COVID-19 pandemic. In L. Castrechini-Franieck (ed.), *Communication with Vulnerable Patients: A Novel Psychological Approach*. London: Routledge, 186–202.

Castrechini-Franieck, L., and Bittner, N., 2022b. T-WAS: Together We Are Strong. In L. Castrechini-Franieck (ed.), *Communication with Vulnerable Patients: A Novel Psychological Approach*. London: Routledge, 155–185.

Foulkes, S.H., and Anthony, E.J., 1990. *Group Psychotherapy: The Psychoanalytic Approach*. 2nd ed. London: Routledge.

Häfele, A., 2009. *Jeder stark im starken Team. 50 Aktionen und Spiele zur Integrationsförderung für Kinder und Jugendliche: [für 6–18 Jahre]*. Mülheim an der Ruhr: Verlag an der Ruhr.

LeCroy, C.W., 1988. Anger management or anger expression. *Residential Treatment for Children & Youth*, 5 (3), 29–39.

Lucas, T., 1988. Holding and holding-on: Using Winnicott's ideas in group psychotherapy with twelve- to thirteen-year-olds. *Group Analysis*, 21 (2), 135–149.

Oaklander, V., 1988. *Windows to Our Children: A Gestalt Therapy Approach to Children and Adolescents*. Highland, NY: Center for Gestalt Development.

Oaklander, V., 2001. Gestalt play therapy. *International Journal of Play Therapy*, 10 (2), 45–55.

Winnicott, D.W., 1960. The theory of the parent-child relationship. *International Journal of Psycho-Analysis*, 41, 585–595.

Winnicott, D.W., et al., eds., 2012/1984. *Deprivation and Delinquency*. Abingdon: Routledge.

Winnicott, D.W., 2014. Aggression in relation to emotional development. In D.W. Winnicott, ed., *Collected Papers: Through Paediatrics to Psycho-Analysis*. London: Routledge, 204–217.

Winnicott, D.W., 2018. The mother-infant experience of mutuality. In *Psycho-Analytic Explorations*. London: Routledge, 251–260.

Woods, J., 1996. Handling violence in child group therapy. *Group Analysis*, 29 (1), 81–98.

Chapter 8

Three different children's groups

From February 2018 to December 2020, three children's groups at three different shared housings for refugees (T, S and B) were run in the city of Stuttgart. The first group (T) took place as a pilot project without us (Leticia and Niko, the group conductors) knowing if and to what extent we would be able to reach the children with such a free-will and easily accessible offer. For the first six months, we were engaged mainly in getting the group up and running. In the first two months, hardly any children came and it was very doubtful that the group would be a success. One time, only a girl came to the group. These initial experiences left us with feelings of hopelessness, powerlessness and emptiness, especially as there were a lot of children living in this particular shelter and they also had a visible presence, hanging out in the courtyard/playground in front of the building in early spring. By sharing these feelings with each other as group leaders, it was possible to give representation to them via a container-contained process (Bion 1984a; Bion 1984b) and we realised that in fact, they belonged to our 'mutuality' process (Winnicott 2018) towards many of the children of our target group. Put more simply, those feelings experienced by us were probably very similar to the ones we presumed the children were familiar with. From this insight, a feeling of connectedness with the children emerged and we gained further strength from it. Our perseverance was rewarded, as by summer 2018, the group was firmly established. At that point, a different religious sponsor from another shared housing for refugees had heard about T-WAS and was clearly in need of a psychosocial group for children and adolescents. Its structure was completely different from that of group T. Situated on the outskirts of the city, this shared housing for refugees was definitely smaller in size and more clearly structured, resembling a small housing estate. When we started group S, right from the beginning, it was clear who among the children wanted to come to us, and they did. Another request from the same sponsor on behalf of a third shared housing for refugees came in at the end of 2018. This time, it was more like an emergency call because the social workers reported a considerable amount of antisocial behaviour, as can be read in chapter 10. Regrettably, we could not offer a third group at that time, since it was beyond our

DOI: 10.4324/9781003466857-11

resources. This request could only be met at the beginning of March 2020 (after completing two years with group T and just before the beginning of the first COVID-19 pandemic lockdown). The third group, group B, was unfortunately run during the severe restrictions of the COVID-19 pandemic, a time during which group work could rarely occur as a face-to-face event, being replaced by telephone calls, as pointed out in chapter 7. The work with group B lasted nine months due to these particular constraints. All in all, in each shared housing for refugees (T and S), there were a total of 80 face-to-face group meetings, whilst just seven at the shared housing for group B. During the COVID-19 pandemic in 2020, there were 16 telephone meetings in both S and B camps and 19 amateur films (as described in chapter 7) were produced. Figure 8.1 illustrates, chronologically, the duration of each group.

I Some parallels between the groups

In all the groups, there was considerable fluctuation during the group formation phase – a trial period with the motto 'Let me see what's going on there'. Even though the dates of the group meetings were pinned up on the door of the group room (in some cases for the whole calendar year), the children always asked at the end of each group if there would be another one. We were able to sense their anxieties and a feeling of distrust which had been created by the deprivations they had encountered in their lives. These emotions can only be processed gradually (Williams 2011).

Another similarity between the groups was that from the very beginning, we were confronted by an ethnic line of conflict, as exemplified in the question 'who plays with chocolate?' – a verbal belittling towards dark-skinned African children, sometimes also accompanied by non-verbal communication, such as furtive derogatory gestures. This should be properly dealt with via games whilst the emotional bond between the group leaders and the participants was still delicate.

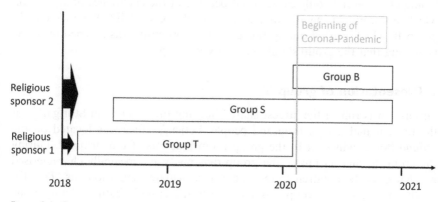

Figure 8.1 Group overview.

It was not by chance that over the formation phase 'batacas', 'card games' and 'being glued to the wall' became the children's favourite games; a mix of a guided cathartic game focused on anger management and two ego-strengthening games focused on dealing with feelings of powerlessness.

Particularly regarding groups T and S, during the group formation phase, lots of children often arrived early, waiting for us in the corridor or in the courtyard before the group started (more as a result of not wanting to lose their control over us). Due to the COVID-19 pandemic, it was not possible for group B to do the same. Over the following phases, this waiting in the corridor turned into a new 'ritual' created by the children themselves, as gradually they became aware of their longing to spend time with us, as well as playing with us and with other children. While waiting, the children used to talk about the group (making plans for it themselves) but also about the eclectic group conductors (their personal profiles). Indeed, several children started notifying us in advance about any possible delays on their part affecting their ability to arrive on time due to family and/or school commitments – an attitude that expressed their sense of responsibility to and acceptance of the group setting, as well as their attachment to the eclectic group conductors. This considerate attitude displayed by the children could be perceived as what Winnicott et al. (2012/1984, p. 86) would probably call 'the capacity for concern' – 'Concern refers to the fact that the individual *cares* or *minds* and both feels and accepts responsibilities'.

The willingness to meet and play with us on a weekly basis emerged as a driving force to transform the separate gender groups into a mixed-gender one. However, some 'trial meetings' were suggested on our part, to assess the boys' and girls' ability to follow the group rules when gathered together. This process differed greatly between the groups, as each group had its own pace of development. For example, the T group became mixed at the beginning of the consolidation phase, whilst group S by the end of the consolidation phase had not yet reached a consensus about merging into a mixed group – the combining of the groups only came about because of the experience of separation which occurred during the first lockdown of the COVID-19 pandemic. In group B, which started during this period, a consensus was reached from the beginning that the group should be a mixed group.

2 Presentation of group T

Group T was run in the largest shared housing for refugees in Stuttgart – at the time, it had over a thousand people. Leticia's office was located on the ground floor, right next to the group room that was at our disposal. During the group formation phase, the group dynamic was repeatedly characterised by chaos, as the children were unable to articulate their thoughts. The disruptive nature of the group was also due to the group's features – a dynamic group matrix could not yet be established. To give an idea of the chaos, towards the end of the farewell timeslot, just after the closing ritual, many children threw chairs on the floor and left the room quickly and screaming – they were simply unable to cope with separation and the act of saying good-bye to us. Gradually, via the ego-relatedness framework encouraged by us, the children were able to find 'external stability' and to develop a group identity – it became possible to establish a dynamic group matrix. In the early part of the consolidation phase, it was increasingly easier for the children to state their feelings in the thumbs-up/thumbs-down check towards the end of the farewell timeslot, which enabled us to move on to creative games focused even more on promoting social interaction. The sports festival was one of the first attempts, shortly before the summer holidays, at introducing community experiences. Both the boys' and girls' groups were invited to play together and the flow of the games was still somewhat orderly. After the summer holidays, we put the possible separation of the groups into boys' and girls' groups up for discussion, partly due to the children's wishes. When a boys' group was scheduled to take place, then girls also came to the group, so we let the boys decide whether the girls could stay or not. The same happened with the girls' group sessions. At the girls' group meetings, the boys tried, on two occasions, to enforce their presence by threating and insulting the girls – a penetrating attitude aiming to push the girls into accepting their presence (an instance of this is mentioned in chapter 9 to illustrate our intervention; see transcript 2). Even though this conflict lasted a period of three months, it was a crucial moment for training 'shared meaning communication'. In time, the children were able to make calculated judgements such as if the boys vote against the girls' presence in the boys' group meeting, there would be an increased chance that the girls would also vote against the boys' presence at the girls' group meetings, which would result in not meeting with us weekly (the girls' and boys' groups alternated, occurring biweekly, respectively). This awareness of the consequences of their actions was a great achievement in the 'shared meaning communication' at this point. From November to December 2018, it was clear that the groups could be mixed, yet the ritual of asking if the girls/boys could stay was kept. This inquiring ritual was a form of self-assurance for the group, as asking reflected the children's awareness that they were and continued to be involved in this conflict resolution process and that they potentially could change back to single-sex groups. This integration process could be clearly seen at the closing party before Christmas in 2018. At their own request, all of the boys and girls spent the closing party cooking, eating together, as well as tidying up and finally giving each other gifts. Following the winter holidays in 2019, the mixed-gender group configuration was no longer an issue. However, there was still no common ground during the rituals. In the bataca fight, boys only challenged boys, and likewise girls only challenged girls, and in the closing circle ('primal scream'), hand-holding between girls and boys was something we repeatedly had to call for as they were unable to do it on their own accord, partly for cultural reasons, thus needing our help. From February onwards, a process of ongoing conflict started in the group. For instance, a birthday celebration in February had to be suddenly cancelled due to the children's behaviour, which descended into anarchy (see birthday celebration guidance notes in chapter 7). In addition, major disruption occurred during the bataca fight in April, which led to two boys being expelled from the group session, after violating the basic group rules. The situation escalated and led to a group rebellion, as detailed further in chapter 9 (see transcript 3). The following weekend, the room opposite the group room (the 'printer room') was vandalised and scribbling on the walls in the corridor increased (Figure 8.2).

These were difficult times. We had to have individual conversations more frequently, and these helped to reduce the out-of-control aggression. Another contributing factor, in our view, that was adding to the tense atmosphere was the fact that we had not yet revealed our involvement in another children's group. The children had seen us together several times, carrying materials like batacas and mashoongas across the yard to put them in our car. So far, we had not invested much energy in clarifying the situation. Aware of this omission, we decided to inform everyone at the next group meeting that there was

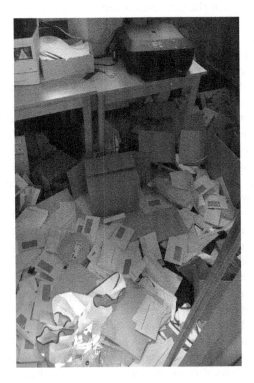

Figure 8.2 Printer room.

a second group of children in another shared housing for refugees. We received many interesting questions from the children about this issue, which were answered transparently.

In the later part of the consolidation phase, the children were able to express their need for more contact and asked for a group excursion. We were unsure whether an all-day excursion would succeed, as the previously described aggressive and impulsive incidents had hardly filled us with confidence, and we communicated this to the children. We therefore informed the children that we would allow an all-day excursion if a group painting project to embellish the corridor could be achieved beforehand. Although the focus was on an intensive all-day get-together on a Saturday, before the all-day excursion, the children perceived the painting project as a punishment. Once more we needed to practice 'shared meaning communication', which took a while to be achieved. This painting project was then reported positively by the press (Reichle, 2019). The result of their efforts became publicly visible and they could feel proud of themselves. The excursion followed, as promised, and this enabled the group to bond together. At the same time, we also started to take pictures of group situations and print them out and hang them in the room in order to raise awareness of the growing history of the children's group. New, younger children were gradually arriving and integrating quickly. Everyone in the shared housing for refugees was aware of the rules of the children's group, and some of the older children took over the function of enforcing them on the new ones. An example of this is lateness – it was clear that one could arrive late but only if this was announced in advance. We also observed that the corridor was not graffitied again after the painting activity. In the farewell phase, the girls then challenged the boys as fighting partners during the bataca rituals, and vice versa. Increasingly, they succeeded in joining hands with each other in the circle during the 'closing ritual', regardless of gender and background – compelling evidence that 'shared meaning communication' could be achieved. Hence, tolerance of diversities improved.

Prior to the Christmas holidays, we also announced the upcoming end of the children's group. The two months before this had focused on ways of constructively helping the children come to terms with their grief associated with the ending of the group. Since most of them had had painful experiences of loss, the aim was for us to frame the farewell as a more positive experience. Remembrance ties through photos and videos, sharing conversations about everyday things, popcorn movie nights, freestyle play and being together without a planned activity marked this phase. Just before the lockdown in late February, we had a moving final celebration where every child received a photo album from us as a gift, with a photo of the 'eclectic group conductors' on the cover (Figure 8.3).

All the children were delighted and hugged us tightly. Just a few minutes after the session ended, some of the children returned to the group room to proudly tell us, 'We are going to have our own children's group now!' – a moving act of self-empowerment on their part that expressed their ability to transform their grief for the better and to focus on the future.

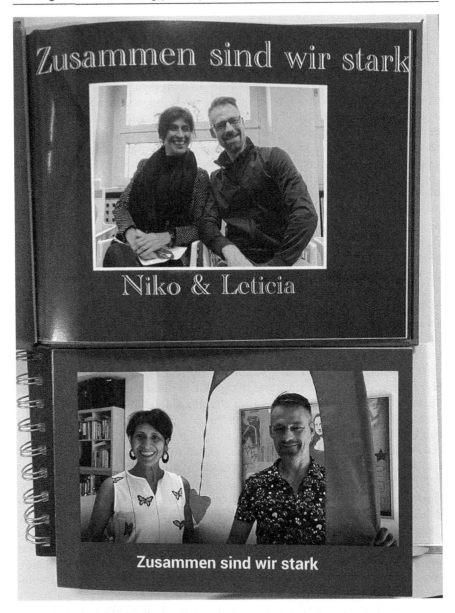

Figure 8.3 Cover of the photo book.

3 Presentation of group S

As with group T, group S started with two groups separated by gender. From the beginning, a real dilemma had to be faced. On two occasions, a few boys did not come to the boys' group as there was an attractive sports programme offered by a male club representative, taking place outdoors at the same time. It started about half an hour before our group and ended correspondingly earlier. We kept making our group rules clear, which stipulated a punctual start and an obligation to stay until the end of the session. In our view, the motto 'Together We Are Strong' mirrored this. We insisted on this motto and so the boys had to decide for themselves which group they wished to join. On an ego-relatedness level, we enabled the boys to experience T-WAS as being a neutral place, where there were no expectations with regards to achievements nor good performance – 'you are welcome as you are!' This neutral space was supposed to be an opportunity for them to engage with creative games and to come willingly. As a result, the leader of the sports programme wanted to join us one time, to understand the reasons why many of the boys were now coming to us and not him. This was an appropriate moment to practise 'shared meaning communication' in the group, according to the motto, 'Better a common solution than a competitive situation'. Thus, a consensus was reached and the sports programme was moved to another day.

The social workers working in the shelter informed us that some children had attracted attention during the summer holiday activities because of their aggressive behaviour. This was also confirmed in the group meetings. However, the expressions of their aggression were not as clearly translated into actions as they were in group T. For instance, during the formation phase, towards the farewell timeslot, in the thumbs-up/thumbs-down questioning, many private conflicts started outside the group setting were unexpectedly raised, which we were, however, unable to work on. We assume that just like when chairs were thrown on the floor in group T, this situation was intended to postpone the group ending, thus, in the same way, avoiding separation. Nevertheless, this situation of being unable to work on the children's needs triggered a strong feeling of powerlessness in us (a counter-transference issue), which was dealt with in our reflection time, after the group. Another kind of aggressive expression related to a form of ritual created by the children themselves. Increasingly, over the course of the group meetings for girls and boys, the participants were observed through the glass doors by the group from the respective opposite-sex and further interruptions occurred in an effort to attract the attention of the 'eclectic group conductors'. They made noises, shook the door or made faces through the viewing window and thus disturbed the group. They were far from wanting to play together; it was more about 'being seen' and 'being in control'. To illustrate the latter, their observations were progressively carried into their next group meetings as a way of trying to get attention, such as, 'But you play more games with the girls!' Indeed, the girls, most of whom were between 10 and 12 years old, tended to be more active in group S than the boys. For example, already after a month, the girls demanded their own games, e.g., musical statues. The final party before the Christmas break was one of the first attempts to introduce community experiences. The needs and requests regarding future plans in the respective boys/girls groups were similar. The celebration was divided into a longer part with games, similar to a regular group session, and a shorter part with a meal together. It was unclear to us whether the bond felt towards us was not yet all that meaningful or whether the topic of separation was unconsciously being avoided by the group. Outwardly, the children showed little emotional response. The different levels of maturity between the boys' and girls' groups became clear to us in 2019. One of the main differences was the way they dealt with the topic of sexuality, which was subject to strong cultural taboos from origin families. The girls had a need to talk about it seriously because of their earlier physical development (e.g., Menarche), despite the fact that Niko, a man, was in the room. They got involved in discussions constructively and could clearly express their thoughts in words, which was not yet feasible for the boys owing to their development and dynamic group matrix. In the case of the boys, the focus was on anger management games. Gradually, it became possible to offer them additional non-ritualised anger management games that required a higher degree of impulse control and social competence as well (this different level of maturity between the girls and boys groups will be addressed in transcript 4 of chapter 9). At the end of 2019, as we informed the group that it would be ending in the summer of 2020, the reactions were marked by surprise and sadness. This triggered the girls' desire to play together with the boys, to enable them to be together with us on a weekly basis, and to intensify the group experiences. January until mid-March 2020 consisted of an ongoing struggle to run the session as a mixed-gender group. However, the puberty-related issues of sexuality along with cultural norms and values remained central to the group's dynamic and frequently triggered conflict within the group. These challenges remained in the foreground for a long period of time, delaying the growth of the group. As eclectic group conductors, we remained more as facilitators in this dynamic matrix. Interestingly, the game of mashoonga was often an effective way of communicating, bringing everyone together. Particularly, the girls showed perseverance and bravely tried to smooth things over, to calm the boys down, for example by saying, '*Yes! We're like a family!*' At one point, when a boy angrily retorted, '*A fake family!*' the girls countered, '*...but still, it's a family!*' This occasion is illustrated in chapter 9 (see transcript 4). In the end, the girls stopped responding, deciding they did not want to play with the boys after all. Then, the last group meeting before the first lockdown due to the COVID-19 pandemic took place, and this was to celebrate Niko's birthday. All the children arranged a surprise, together with the help of Leticia, and everyone kept Niko in the dark about it. The children received the key to the group room and independently got themselves there and hid in the dark room in order to scare Niko when he unlocked the door. Despite the conflicts among them, they did in fact manage to do this. A new impulse was created; however, it could not be properly managed, owing to the abrupt lockdown. A two-month separation until we could re-establish contact with the children followed, as outlined in chapter 7. Consequently, the end of the group was planned to be postponed until December, so that we could perhaps meet again and end the group properly. In September and October 2020, we had five meetings where the focus was on playing together. The meetings were large, with more than 20 children, full of joy and excitement at seeing each other again. Mixed-gender games were not an issue anymore. From November onwards, lockdown restrictions applied again and we returned to phone calls, letters and films as a way of keeping in touch until December (see chapter 7). At the last meeting in early December, we were able to say goodbye to two children at the same time and give them a photo album as a gift, with the photo of the 'eclectic group conductors' on the cover, as we did in the farewell of group T (see Figure 8.3). Regrettably, in the meantime, some of the children had moved away without us having the opportunity to say goodbye to them. In the end, this situation left us with a feeling of emptiness and also doubts as to whether we were achieving any-thing. Perhaps we had failed to achieve our goals in part because we were unable to keep providing a stable environment based on ego-relatedness. The farewell phase, which is based on family events and encouraging the imagi-nation, had ultimately failed. We did try to assist the children during the lockdowns, and we achieved this, but only partially.

4 Presentation of group B

The same as with the groups T and S, we scheduled gender-separated groups and started with the girls' group, which was immediately attended by 12 girls and was intense. Our first meeting was also the last one before the first lock-down due to the COVID-19 pandemic. Having hardly seen the children in real life made the long lockdown phase from March to September very chal-lenging. In particular, we had not even had a meeting with the boys and had to get to know each other through films. Similar to what was described for group S, group B underwent the interplay of keeping in touch through phone calls, letters with photos and films of us – contact in 'digital mode'. For instance, the first film was a guessing game about us. In September and October, when we were able to meet the children again (and finally met the boys in person for the first time), a willingness to be with us quickly devel-oped, along with a sense of togetherness among the children. The children showed a great longing and desire to get to know each other, especially in a structured setting. None of the girls or boys questioned playing together. After two years, we also performed well together as a couple, and the children were able to perceive this from the films as well. The second lockdown came at the beginning of November and we returned to 'digital mode'. In Decem-ber, we met the children for the last time in groups of two to say farewell. Therefore, we had few opportunities to create a community over the course of three quarters of a year and eight group meetings. The bond we had with the children was repeatedly disrupted. We failed to achieve our main goal of promoting competence in everyday conflict resolution through playful methods. On the animation level, however, we succeeded in building up the bond and keeping it in parts. In view of this, the group work was concluded at the end of the year. The farewell followed the same procedure as with group S. Many children arrived on time, signed up for the schedule, respected the short playing time and the AHA formula, and showed commitment whilst visibly having fun. The AHA formula is an abbreviation in German for distance, hygiene and everyday life with a mask. It advises a minimum distance of 1.5 metres from other people be kept, hygiene rules be observed, such as thorough hand washing, and a mask, preferably FFP2, be worn in everyday life (Presse- und Informationsamt der Bundesregierung n.d.).

To our surprise, the resonance of our films was much more positive and lively in face-to-face conversations than by phone call. We gave everyone a gift of a photo card of the 'eclectic group conductors'.

5 Some personal observations

As pointed out in chapter 2, a relationship with a child is based on face-to-face contact, and being in contact is characterised by the five basic channels of human perception that have shaped us since birth: sight, hearing, touch, smell and taste (Oaklander 2001). Should one or more of these channels fail, then the representation of what we have perceived is affected – the intensity of contact is diminished. This kind of contact was only possible in group T throughout the period of two years in face-to-face meetings. Family-like experiences and encouraging the imagination, the pillars of the farewell phase, led to an intensification of relationships in the group, to a feeling of belonging, to the achievement of 'shared meaning communication', and to the strengthening of resilience. It would have been great to have similar experiences with groups S and B, but owing to the COVID-19 pandemic, the farewell phase failed in later groups, and this led to a gap in supporting a secure framework of ego-relatedness in-group. Reflecting on the development of the consolidation phase regarding groups S and T, in group S the group dynamic was strongly marked by the topic of whether boys and girls would be able to be in a group together. Conversely, being together had a greater significance in group T, particularly once the boys managed to get their request for a mixed-gender group accepted. They succeeded in doing so through forceful, persistent behaviour towards the girls, i.e., coming to every group session and then refusing to leave the room, a 'ritual' which lasted for almost three months. From a symbolic point of view, in group T, the children were able to make use of their transitional space to playfully express their aggression and love, therefore achieving 'shared meaning communication'. Their aggression (or their forceful, persistent behaviour) was directed towards a common objective – being together (their love). However, in group S, the children were unable to make full use of their transitional space.

They remained stuck in their dilemma, in which their aggression (mutual insults) was directed at avoiding unity (most likely due to fear) instead of towards love. The first and last community action displayed by group S, namely Niko's surprise birthday party, clearly revealed that the children indeed needed more time, more space and strong emotional support from us (the eclectic group conductors) in modes of relatedness towards the development of their dynamic group matrix. It is true that the production of animated films can be regarded as modes of trying to remain connected to the children; however, our relationships could not deepen in the same way as via face-to-face contact. This was even more the case for group B. Nevertheless, it was surprising to us to learn that it was also possible to start relationships through a 'digital mode'. After all, up to this point, we had had no experience of using this kind of approach to group work with children.

References

Bion, W.R., 1984a. *Learning from Experience*. London: Maresfield.

Bion, W.R., 1984b. *Second Thoughts: Selected Papers on Psychoanalysis*. London: Routledge.

Oaklander, V., 2001. Gestalt play therapy. *International Journal of Play Therapy*, 10 (2), 45–55.

Presse- und Informationsamt der Bundesregierung, n.d. *Die 'AHA-Regeln' im neuen Alltag*. www.bundesregierung.de/breg-de/themen/coronavirus/die-aha-regeln-im-neuen-alltag-1758514.

Reichle, S., 2019. Zusammen sind wir stark. *Stuttgarter Wochenblatt*, 10 July, 2.

Williams, A., 2011. *Working with Street Children: An Approach Explored*. Lyme Regis: Russell House.

Winnicott, D.W., *et al.*, eds., 2012/1984. *Deprivation and Delinquency*. Abingdon: Routledge.

Winnicott, D.W., 2018. The mother-infant experience of mutuality. In *Psycho-Analytic Explorations*. London: Routledge, 251–260.

Chapter 9

Direct challenges from children to eclectic group conductors

As referred to in chapter 1, coping with antisocial tendencies (and/or behaviour) implies being faced with aggression. The more the eclectic group conductors are able to offer an ego-relatedness group framework, by providing the child with ego support, the more the children will display expressions of aggression, and the eclectic group conductors should be able to deal with their repeated attacks (Winnicott et al. 2012/1984; Woods 1996), and it will not be the case that the provision of ego support will lead to the children getting calmer. What kinds of aggression might be displayed within a group setting will depend exclusively on the dynamic group matrix of each group, and no effective responses can be provided for how one should behave in such situations. To illustrate, four challenging situations (four of many) are presented and discussed in this chapter through four group transcripts, as they were a direct challenge to the work of T-WAS. They are ordered chronologically from February 2018 to February 2020. The first scenario refers to the very beginning of T-WAS, exactly at the point when the eclectic group conductors were trying to find their feet. The case describes an experience of miscommunication that triggered the leaders' awareness of the co-existing variables that may exert both external and internal influences upon leadership performance. The second and third transcripts refer to two meetings of group T, the former at the end of the formation phase and the latter in the middle of the consolidation phase. The fourth one refers to a group S meeting at the end of the consolidation phase. All transcripts presented here were based on our vivid memories of the group meetings, or according to Bion (1965) based on the representations of our emotional experiences triggered by our contact with the children, as well as with each other. We never recorded a group session. Therefore, occasionally the transcripts might lack detail, which may have an influence on their coherence. Each transcript is subdivided into a description of the current group context, the progress transcript, the eclectic group conductors' evaluation and concluding remarks. More precisely, the eclectic group conductors' evaluation covers the clarification of possible individual procedures, including the personal understanding of protocol for each member of the eclectic group. In this manner, the reader may vividly experience their individual perspectives. Our explanatory thoughts during the progress of

DOI: 10.4324/9781003466857-12

the group session are all written in italics. Emphasis will be placed on the relationship among the children themselves, between the children and the eclectic group conductors, and between the eclectic group conductors themselves, rather than on method.

1 Transcription 1: Miscommunication

Context: this transcription refers to a group meeting in the very early stages of the work of T-WAS. At that time, we had not started writing transcripts yet, nor had we adopted the four basic procedures (see chapter 5), and nor had we thought about the influences on leadership performance (see also chapter 5). This transcript refers to a boys' group that took place fortnightly. A total of ten boys took part in the group. We are unable to remember their names and ages.

Progress: The group started with a 'big round' of the bataca fight. Some children were still not used to the game; thus its rules were occasionally infringed. At this point, we just reminded the children about the rules without applying any sanctions; after all, they were still in the learning process. A new boy arrived late. He had never heard about the 14 rules before (see chapter 5 for more details on these rules). Indeed, at that time, we used to only address the rules verbally at the beginning of the group meeting. During the bataca round, Niko pointed out the first rule again, namely *'only speak German'*, as he believed this new boy was talking in his mother tongue. The group was quite restless, and it was difficult to notice everything that was going on. Suddenly, Niko yelled and asked the new boy to leave the group immediately. The children and Leticia were surprised with Niko's sanction, and whilst the boy left the room, with tears in his eyes, there was some disruption and the children became unsettled. Niko explained that he had already given him three warnings.

Although Leticia was unable to understand what was going on and the reasons why Niko was so harsh on the new boy, she decided not to contest his decision, even though she did not agree with it at all (Ballhausen-Scharf et al. 2021). Indeed, this could also have been a counter-transferential response on Niko's part.

Niko then suggested a second bataca fight, a 'big round'. Leticia remarked that the children might not want to do a second round and suggested playing another game. Niko did not listen to Leticia and led a second round by himself. The children became more restless.

Niko's aim in doing the second round was to allow the children to become aware of their anger, as referred to by Oaklander (1988, p. 211), in order for them to recognise its origin, which was in fact the incident which had just happened in the group. Leticia's point of view was quite different from Niko's, as according to her, the children were distressed due to the puzzling situation with the new boy, and therefore, the group's participants were more in need of a 'container-contained interaction' instead of a cathartic one. At this point, the eclectic group conductors worked entirely separately, according to different approaches, but still showing respect to each other – the latter sets up the main path leading to the achievement of 'shared meaning communication' between them.

Although the miscommunication between the eclectic group conductors was noticed by everyone, the group started playing a card game. During the thumbs-up/thumbs-down feedback, a quarter of the children gave a thumbs-down, i.e., one of them felt undervalued and others felt that the group lacked creativity that day.

Leticia was also unhappy with the group session and left the group with a question in her mind: how many boys would come on the next meeting?

1.1 Eclectic group conductors' evaluation

After the group meeting, Leticia asked Niko for a quick chat about that particular session. During the conversation, it became clear that Niko was not aware of his oppressive attitude during the group session, yet he confessed that he was not in a good mood that day. Leticia expressed how this group session had been exhausting, as a lot of the group time was focused on playing bataca, which may be good for the expression of anger, but not good enough for processing it via a 'container-contained interaction'. A cathartic release of emotion on a physical level does not bring symbolisation; it does not help in transforming beta into alpha elements, nor does it support the development of the reflection ('thought-thinking apparatus' – Bion 1962). As we suspected, the children's poor evaluation of the group on that particular day could be attributed to our miscommunication. From this group meeting onwards, we started adopting the four basic procedures – 1) mutual understanding communication, 2) regular professional exchange, 3) conscious handling of conflicts, and 4) supervision – as well as reflecting on the influences upon leadership performance. We have learnt that these are crucial for being able to offer a successful, secure and neutral space for the children. We also started to write down the 14 rules and make them accessible.

1.2 Concluding remarks

Regarding our different perspectives while leading the group, despite them, we kept playing with the children rather than dwelling on our differences and engaging in a discussion or a dispute. Our attitude may have been perceived by the children as a new, active approach in dealing with diversities once our differences had become abundantly clear to them. Conversely, in terms of the counter-transference issues raised within the group, as noted by Foulkes and Anthony (1990), when Niko expelled the new boy from the group in a tyrannical way, he might have been assuming the authoritarian role reserved for the male archetypal figure (the father), while Leticia's silence and submission would have corresponded to the female archetypal figure (the mother). At this point, both remarks may and should be reflected upon and considered. It is not about making a decision based on 'either this... or that'. Rather, it is about identifying possibilities based on the idea of 'both/and'. The eclectic group conductors should also be able to practise the principle of 'shared meaning communication' in their reflections, otherwise they will fail in passing this on to the children.

2 Transcription 2: Pushy boys

Context: This transcription refers to the work of T-WAS at the end of the group formation phase. It was a girls' group day in shared housing for group T that took place fortnightly on Wednesdays from 5:30 to 7:00 pm. In total, the following children were present: seven boys, including Be (aged 12), San (aged 12), Sah (aged 13), Sal (aged 13), Ai (aged 10), Si (aged 8) and Sol (aged 11), and three girls, including S (aged 10), H (aged 8), and Sha (aged 13). At that time, the dynamic group matrix (Foulkes and Anthony 1990) of both the girls' and boys' groups was still marked by an unconscious desire to merge the groups. However, no structured thought process of negotiation had been initiated thus far, as their desire did not have a mental representation, rather it was instead experienced in action (more details about group T's dynamic matrix are available in chapter 8).

Progress: Leticia opened the group room at 5 pm whilst singing a Brazilian song, and the children started coming into the group room. When Niko arrived, at 5:15 pm, a couple of children were already sitting on their chairs in a circle. Then, Be suggested the group start immediately. Leticia stopped singing and pointed out that the group was supposed to start at 5.30 pm and that they would wait until then, as other children might yet also arrive. Leticia started singing again. Meanwhile the group was relatively quiet.

A quiet moment triggered by the singing approach as described in chapter 7.

Niko took advantage of this moment of calm to snack on a loaf of bread with red peppers. Then, Sal tried to convince Niko to start the group by playing something, though initially Niko could not hear him.

Here, for the first time, the penetrating force that will characterise the dynamic group matrix of this meeting can be seen. By trying to convince Niko to play something, Sal was also imposed Be's wish on Leticia – to start the group before 5.30 pm.

Then, Sal asked Leticia whether would listen to him. Leticia was aware of what Sal was trying to do and she answered, 'Sorry, I am singing now!' Sal's reaction to Leticia's response was to make fun of Niko's name, as 'Niko' in Arabic means 'fuck'.

This information is true, yet at that time, we were unsure about it. Nevertheless, it is clear that Sal's aggressive energy was being expressed in the group setting, in quite an intrusive manner.

Leticia laughed and started telling Niko that everything went together very nicely: the meaning of his name together with eating the red pepper. Niko was not able to understand Leticia's (erotic) joke straightaway. Then, Leticia teased Niko by saying that his fantasies/imagination were not so great and she laughed; Niko finally understood her comments.

At this point, it was not clear to us why Leticia had this 'daydreaming' as termed by Cassorla (2018 , p. 8). Why did 'eating the red pepper' spontaneously emerge as an erotic image in her mind? In any case, Leticia's joke also had penetrating features, like Sal's one.

Apart from this, Leticia and Niko started talking about dressing up for Halloween and other things planned for the group, so that their attention was focused on organising the next group meetings, while they were waiting for the group to start – like when 'dad' and 'mum' are busy, planning things for their children. Then, the group started to become restless and an abrupt physical confrontation between two boys broke out, as one said to the other, 'I am fucking your mother!'

Once more, an intrusive, erotic verbalisation and image emerged, now in a new, more concrete context.

Niko intervened at this point and separated the two by saying that if they wanted to continue fighting, they would have to do this in the courtyard and not in the group room, which they actually did, accompanied by all the other five boys. Then, Niko went after them and tried to calm them down. After a couple of minutes, everyone came back into the group room.

At the beginning, Niko tried to give the boys the chance to reflect on their behaviour instead of acting as an arbiter; yet, the boys were still unable to reflect on what had happened. They were very much in need of an arbiter (or a father figure that could intervene in the 'mother to be fucked by another one' scenario).

Nevertheless, the group became more restless, i.e., Leticia had to address the group in a raised voice so that Niko was able to talk to the group. It was exactly 5.30 pm when we started the group. Niko reminded all the children that today was a girls' group meeting. We both agreed on how to proceed and we let the three girls decide whether the boys could stay or not. However, this decision had to be applied to all the boys without exception – a dilemma for Sha, since her brother (Be) was one of the seven boys. At this moment, Be raised the question as to why there had to be two separate groups, one for girls and another for boys – why couldn't we just be one mixed-gender group?

A rather intriguing and accurate question on the part of Be, which we, as eclectic group conductors, totally failed to address, owing to the chaotic scenario brought about by the fight between the two boys. Indeed, it was the first time that a verbal representation of the unconscious desire to merge the groups had been provided. Once again, Be's complaint can also be perceived as 'penetrating', like the previous one. Nevertheless, this time, the aim was to bring the groups together, which can also be understood as the expression of a positive form of aggression, as referred to by Blom (2006) and Oaklander (1988), since it was an attempt to reach a homeostasis outcome. From Winnicott's (1960) point of view, this may illustrate the interplay between aggression and love – the expression of primary aggression in-group.

Meanwhile, one of the boys involved in the fight kept speaking in his mother tongue, despite Niko warning him three times. Leticia then identified his sanction. He left the group room in an angry manner, i.e., insulting the whole group and by placing a chair on the table and then hitting the chair with the palm of his hand.

Clearly a non-verbal expression of his aggressive energy, triggered by the feeling of frustration – a cathartic manner for trying to achieve homeostasis as referred to in Gestalt therapy. His attitude may be related to the instances of 'Niko = fuck' or 'eating a red pepper' or 'I am fucking your mother', yet this time, the aggressive energy was clearly and consciously expressed towards the group conductors and in-group.

Following this, we asked all the boys to leave the room so that the girls could make their decision without feeling under pressure, because of the boys' presence, but mainly due to issues concerning sibling loyalty. When all the boys were finally outside, the girls' voted in favour of being on their own. When we shared the girls' decision with the boys, they got quite angry. As Niko opened the door and asked them to please leave us to start the group, they simply poured back into the room. The boys then started a chorus of 'We boys stay, we boys stay!' They repeated this loudly and persistently, building up their anger.

The tension was high and although we were perplexed, our reaction was not to suppress the boys but rather to wait to assess the situation more accurately.

Next, they started climbing onto the windowsills and the tables in order to hide and so on, whilst we tried to figure out what was going on, while trying to keep cool. This dragged on for a good five minutes, perhaps even ten, and was exhausting for everyone. The girls sat there quietly and quite patiently for most of the time. The situation escalated to the point of overflowing outside the group setting. For example, a father came into the hallway and spoke briefly to Leticia, explaining that he had sent a boy (the one who needed to leave the group) away from the window from the courtyard side. Hence, even from the outside, an uneasy situation was noticed.

As a result, we began thinking separately whether we should seek external help, like the security guard at the gate of the shared housing for refugees. Following this, we started sharing our thoughts, besides the products of our imaginations triggered by our feelings of helplessness combined with the fear of failing. Being able to be in contact with these feelings and to support each other helped us to find the trust in ourselves as eclectic group conductors and further to allow the boys to make use of their transitional space to express playfully their aggression and love. From this moment on, the boys calmed down and stopped their actions, at least in the group room.

In the end, the boys relented little by little, but they were so persistent even after leaving the room that we kept the door locked. This went on for another 5–10 minutes, during which, the boys knocked on the door and the window from outside, sat on the windowsills outside, and jumped up briefly and then jumped down again. When we were finally alone with the girls, we apologised for taking so long to start the group meeting and informed them that we had one hour left. Then, we started playing relatively quickly. Everyone seemed to be quite clear about the programme: a big round of the bataca fight, the card game and then a girl would be glued to the wall. At this meeting, the winner of the card game was S, a girl who had come to the group for the first time and hardly spoke any German. Everything ran quite smoothly.

During the gluing game, Niko complained of pain in his hand and Leticia made fun of him, referring to him as 'an old man'. Both were enjoying the joke. Then, Sha got bitter and started moaning.

Once more, a 'penetrating' reaction, now on the part of the girls arose, and was directed straight towards the eclectic group conductors – quite a similar situation to when the two boys started fighting while the group conductors were chatting.

Sha remarked that Niko had gold teeth and Niko teased her with a joke by saying, 'Why don't you marry me? I'll die soon, and then you can inherit the gold!'

A rather dangerous joke on Niko's part, as the topic of marriage has enormous moral value in the culture of these children.

Sha responded in an offended, yet flirtatious, manner by persuading Niko to commit to giving her a gift as a form of apology. Niko agreed and made a commitment to bring Sha a gift.

The 'penetrating' force appears again, now masked by flirting. Although Leticia did not agree with Niko's commitment, as according to her, this should be worked out and not acted out, she remained silent.

Meanwhile S was glued to the wall. Then, we took photos. For the last ten minutes, we played music. Sha picked the music and Niko took out a flow ring. The ring has a stainless-steel mesh that can be rolled along the arm and passed from arm to arm. The game went well. Leticia picked up a few dance moves from Niko, originating from the Bavarian Shoe-slapper knee dance. Both clapped their own thighs and shoes and gave whoops, so they clearly had fun whilst dancing. Sha reacted angrily once more and tried to stop the dance by choosing music from her home country.

It is worth mentioning that due to the loud music while we were dancing, some boys started disturbing us again with shouts from outside. They also jumped onto the windowsills. So, the 'penetrating' forces came from both sides: in-group via Sha and via the boys outside.

During the feedback round, everyone signalled they were happy with this meeting, despite all the initial disruption. Then, when the girls left the group room, one of the seven boys quickly tried to enter the room again, but Niko energetically prevented him from doing so and used his arm to obstruct him. Another boy remarked that the group 'sucked'.

2.1 Eclectic group conductors' evaluation

Interestingly, after this group session, during the group conductors' reflection, Niko referred to the following topics: 'macho' culture, the connection between aggressiveness and sexuality (pre-rape), the differences between males and females, and the armed forces, as illustrated below.

Niko's thoughts: With respect to the context, the preliminary consideration on my part favoured the gender-specific separation of the children's groups. From a professional point of view, psychosocial children's groups should take gender development into account as a prominent category. This was my professional understanding. I perceived myself as part of the cultural-pedagogical development in western societies of always highlighting one's own identity in gender-segregated groups, which of course can also include non-binary aspects of self-attribution. This separation of genders is something that is rarely found at school, as a co-educational place of education, and likewise is presumably also given little attention in families. Two things are important here with regards to the children's groups. Firstly, there is the acquisition of information about the values and norms of the host society, about 'the field' in which the children gain orientation, by the eclectic group conductors making it available for performing the work of translation. Secondly, there is the idea of taking the pressure off 'refugee children' as a unified group and thereby stimulating and supporting discussions within the migrant field, by the eclectic group conductors trying to understand the girls' opinions, as well as those of the boys, and encouraging them to exchange their thoughts and to model this exchange on an equal level. For example, the idea that girls are allowed to exchange ideas in girls' groups, a common idea in our cultural self-image, was brought to the foreground by us and was 'defended' against the boys' need to 'be in charge'. The clear support from us as eclectic group conductors helped the girls to learn to hold their own position and the behaviour that I displayed in standing firm during the confrontation with the boys (I did not let myself become their plaything) was certainly an important signal. Ultimately, it was also a very real and understandable signal; a relationship experience that makes concepts related to values tangible: as a man, I accept the position of girls who want their own space for development.

In the German-speaking, western society, boys as well as girls are granted so-called trial behaviour during puberty. In confrontation with a girl, this space emerges, which I would like to call 'flirting as a testing field'. In the protected setting of the children's group, the challenging behaviour of the markedly teenage Sha is to be understood as such when she abruptly makes statements about, for example, my gold teeth. My no less challenging response on the topic of a 'marriage proposal', mixed with the idea of a 'perspective of economic gain' is to be regarded within the framework of the eclectic group conductors. Presumably, if I had been the sole group leader, I would have responded differently. Leticia was, however, present and thus able to take the girl's side and 'push me back' again, supporting the girl in her empowerment. In this way, my position of male power (old, rich, offering and luring) was transformed into the position of male responsibility (taking age difference into account, respecting boundaries, ensuring balance).

Leticia's thoughts: When the two boys started their fight before the group began, my idea at that moment was to offer them the mashoongas as a transitional object, then they could express their anger in a playful manner whilst receiving our support for their anger. However, the group had not started yet and this could have been confusing for all the children, as we were still at the end of the formation phase. Indeed, the boys were more in need of an arbiter and/or 'a father'.

I fully appreciate Niko's thoughts, yet in my opinion, his thoughts strongly represent the daunting challenges posed by the environment for the children (especially for vulnerable ones) in dealing with polarities. In this case, for Niko, it was quite important to maintain the gender polarities. Psychologically, what caught my attention most was the constant presence of this 'penetrating force' coming from both sides: from the children's side and from mine through my erotic joke – a clear counter-transferential issue, as outlined by Foulkes and Anthony (1990). One should keep in mind that due to the precarious home lives of these pre-pubescent children (families being agglomerated in small rooms in the shared housing for refugees), they have undoubtedly been exposed to some kinds of awful experiences. For instance, most of their parents did not have their own bedrooms nor did they conduct their sex lives in private, which implies that probably several children might have already been confronted by their parents' sexual activities. Hence, it is more than reasonable to assume that the children will have made use of the group's transitional space to work through their ambiguous and blurred feelings (aggression and love) about sexuality, and, of course, it is expected that this would be expressed in an aggressive and 'penetrating' manner. I particularly experienced 'this force' not as an attempt to dominate, but rather as a cry for help (Winnicott et al. 2012/1984).

2.2 Concluding remarks

One must keep in mind that, despite all the disruption, at no time was the aggression aimed at hurting anyone, not even when the two boys started a physical fight; otherwise, Niko would not have been successful in stopping it. The 'penetrating force' was a movement directed towards achieving a change, rather than destroying something – realising this form of communication is directly related to the ability of the group conductors in dealing with in-group aggression (Woods 1996). As a matter of fact, this force was the means by which the children were not only testing our endurance in dealing with their aggressive energy and/or primary aggression, but were also gaining confidence in their relationship with us.

Concerning the eclectic group conductors' thoughts, despite our different points of view, we did work as a team and the moments of joking between us were the link that connected us. We made use of our transitional space to find each other in this chaos and at that moment, the children were able to perceive us as a unit, as well as individuals. A remarkable moment demonstrating this happened during the disruption when we, the eclectic group conductors, were overcome by our personal fears, yet trusted each other to share them. By doing so, we were able to find our unity and increased our resources to be able to carry on, while enduring the children's attacks. This very situation had a positive impact on the boys, otherwise they would not have left the group room on their own. It is exactly this that represents the value of the eclectic group conductors as a resource.

3 Transcription 3: Rebellion

Context: This transcription refers to the work of T-WAS in the middle of the consolidation phase in the shared housing for refugees of group T. It is a mixed-gendered group that meets weekly on Wednesdays from 5:30 pm to 7:00 pm. In total, the following children participated in the group on this day: 15 boys, Ae (aged 12), Ai (aged 10), San (aged 12), Sah (aged 13), Ko (aged 11), All (aged 13), E (aged 7), Be (aged 12), Si (aged 8), Su (aged 11), Ya (aged 12), Sal (aged 13), K (aged 10), Y (aged 11) and Der (aged 10), and seven girls, Ha (aged 11), Di (aged 9), Shi (aged 10), An (aged 11), Sha (aged 13), Hi (aged 9) and S (aged 10).

As mentioned in the previous chapter, this transcript refers to a time when we were facing a process of ongoing conflict in the group. The day before, when we were rushing to get to the shared housing for refugees for group S, we met Ae, who asked us where we were going to, and we answered him briefly that we were running another children's group in another shared housing for refugees. A couple of hours before the start of the group meeting in question here, Leticia had met several children. Sah informed her that yesterday, the children had supposed that there would be a group meeting. Then, when they saw the dates of the group meetings pinned up on the door of the group room, they realised they were wrong. Today, the sheet with the dates of the group meetings had been torn away by someone.

Progress: The group room was full of children (N = 22); four were in the group for the first time. We started the group punctually at 5.30 pm. Before the starting ritual, we chatted about different matters, i.e., whether Leticia had ever met a Brazilian football player, and whether Paris is a beautiful city or not. Then, Ai drew a silhouette of the Eiffel Tower in the air. The talk turns to Notre-Dame, which has been half burnt down. The mood was friendly and calm. As the group was quite large, far more of our attention was required, and so a small round of bataca was better. Leticia and Niko took the lead and fought first.

Then Be challenged Sah, but they started messing around, i.e., hitting more than they were allowed to, lifting their legs up and carrying out block hits.

From this moment on, the group meeting started to descend into chaos.

Once the bataca fights were over, Sah announced, while grinning broadly, that he had to leave, as he had another appointment. San wanted to follow him, then the new group members, who still did not know the rule that whoever joins the group must stay until the end, wanted to leave as well. Then, Leticia called Sha to a face-to-face conversation in her office. Leticia made it clear to him that he was welcome to leave the group, yet as she was suspicious of the motives behind him wanting to leave, her trust in him began to wane. Leticia made it clear to him that her aim for this face-to-face chat was to share her thoughts (about him) with him, so that he could keep trusting her. As a result, Sha then said to Leticia that he had decided to stay.

This is an approach from TICA (Castrechini-Franieck, 2022 , p. 29) – 'the emphasis is on creating a transitional space that may allow a new experience in communicating in relationships with others'.

Meanwhile, one of the new members often yelled whilst pretending to cry in an exaggerated manner. Another of the new members fell down together with Su, while pushing a wooden chair with impetus into the bataca fight, even though Leticia had already given them two warnings beforehand. Inevitably, the third warning came and these two boys were to be kicked out. In protest at the eclectic group conductors' decision, they started banging on the door, opening it, and slamming it again and again.

In such an atmosphere, it was impossible to conduct group activities in a safe manner. We decided then to lock the door, not only to stop the repetitive disruption, but above all, to protect the group setting.

Unable to come inside the room, both the boys started throwing rubbish from outside through the cracked windows.

Once more to protect the group setting, the windows were closed. The group was already in chaos.

Si and E started to fall out, as the former felt provoked by the latter. Leticia tried to talk to Si privately, and to calm him down, she told him that she had missed his presence at the last meeting; yet due to the strong manifestation of his aggressive energy, he could not be reached. At the same time, the remaining friend of the new group member started making even more intense noises like a 'cry-baby'. Meanwhile, things became even more chaotic outside, as the two 'kicked out' boys called the security guards at the gate of the shared housing for refugees. They complained to them that we, the eclectic group conductors, were keeping other children locked in a room against their will. Suddenly, the security knocked on the door of the group room. We were able to notice them through the viewing window of the door. The security consisted of a man and a woman, and they were accompanied by the two boys. Leticia left the group room, while Niko stayed with the group. The security wanted to know what was going on because both the children had been 'complaining' about children being mistreated. Leticia then explained to the security that it was a weekly children's group and that everything was okay. She also explained that both the boys who had complained had just had to leave the group because they had not followed the rules and were near to hurting someone. The two guards then left.

From this moment on, the worst part of the chaotic phase started.

Several children in the group room started throwing the plastic chairs on top of each other in the centre of the circle, while yelling. E suddenly threw one of his rubber shoes at Leticia. Batacas were fetched to be played with in the wrong manner.

Repeatedly, we had to take the batacas off the children and bring them to safety by saying, 'No, that's not being used now'.

The children did not/could not listen to us, and the use of a louder voice, as suggested by Franck (1997), was useless. Here, a Gestalt therapy approach would not work, as the aggressive energy had been greatly expressed via aggressive acts upon us and on the group as well. It was a real expression of psychological chaos that needed to be contained. Therefore, a conscious and controlled response of silence on our part (in the sense of being persistent) was quite possibly the most powerful form of communication between us and the children. However, this should be done by using body language as a means of expressing our feelings. That is why we decided to turn our chairs with our backs to the group and maintained this position for about 20 minutes! We could not sit with our backs to the group all the time. We did it in such a way that we could intervene if necessary, for example if there was a risk of injury. During this process, we kept on looking into each other's eyes while questioning ourselves as to whether we would be able to achieve 'a shared meaning communication' with the children by using this approach, since the situation was quite frightening. Via eye contact, we mutually supported each other and once more, we acted 'with one voice' as eclectic group conductors, like we did in transcription 2. In this manner, the safe space within the group, as well as its containment function, could be restored (Ballhausen-Scharf et al. 2021; Lehle 2018; Woods 1996).

Lastly, at some stage, communication between us and the children took place. Their aggressive energy level dropped. Sal began to pile up the chairs and Ae also helped him, whilst a new space, a new mood emerged. Half the group sat quietly; the rest continued to be restless, though at this point, it was possible to address the group. Then, Leticia said she was sorry for what had happened.

Her words were addressed to everyone, yet those who had conducted themselves in a more constructive manner might have felt that they were being addressed.

Leticia added, 'Next week, we'll have our group again, then we might think about who will be allowed or not allowed to take part in it!' Following this, Niko announced that those who wanted to leave the group room could do so now, and those who wanted to stay to talk about the situation were welcome to stay. Most of the children left the group room. All the girls, Sal, Y and Ko stayed.

This approach appealed again to those who really wanted to stay with us. At this point, our impulsive inner reaction was to not allow the children who had displayed antisocial tendencies to come back to the group. This was a strong counter-transferential reaction on our part, triggered by the recently experienced chaos, which afterwards was fully discussed, reviewed and re-evaluated in the course of our reflection time, and, of course, the children were allowed to come back to future group meetings.

Then, the remaining children all reported what had happened as we turned our chairs around. Talking about our emotional experiences of the chaos helped all of us to put these experiences into words and into further representations of them, which was quite therapeutic. As a result, we were able to briefly plan the painting project, i.e., no more than 12 children would be allowed on the project. All the children agreed. Niko complimented the children for staying calm and for attending. Leticia got some lollies from her office, a soothing gesture. We ended the group with the closing ritual.

3.1 Eclectic group conductors' evaluation

Niko's thoughts: This experience was very intense and put my ability to surrender to the test. A paradoxical situation was created, so to speak, with the clearly communicated withdrawal of the two group conductors. Rather than act in response to the aggression more activity – a reaction that is always accompanied by the inner illusion of control over a situation – I trusted myself to the shared idea of leading in silence, without knowing whether it would work. Actually, I was unsure whether the bond with the group would be able to take the strain, especially due to the dynamic of the new boys in the group.

Leticia's thoughts: This experience took me back to a fight between two prisoners in the withdrawal station in the therapeutic community (Castrechini-Franieck 2022). The regular procedure in that case was to isolate both prisoners in their cells, while the others were not given any explanation about what was going on, remaining in a chaotic situation and quite restless – an occasion susceptible to triggering a rebellion. Then, contrary to the rules, I decided to run an impromptu group session with all the 16 male prisoners to talk about what had just happened, despite all the risk of them starting a rebellion with me there. This common sense approach of offering the prisoners a neutral space for their thoughts in order to put them at ease was similar to the one I had experienced in this group session with the children. Despite their aggressiveness, I was still very much interested in finding ways to communicate with them. An image of being in a maternity ward, full of babies crying all at the same time popped into my mind. What might be done in such a situation? The willingness to be there, even if in silence, seemed to me to be the accurate approach to contain such chaos. At no point did I feel afraid of the children's aggression; I was, rather, worried about the consequences I would have to face the next day owing to the children's report to the security guards – a genuine occurrence, since I had to explain why we had kept the children locked in a room to state child welfare authorities. The fear of having to abruptly interrupt the group meetings was what scared me the most – what may clearly be perceived as an alpha element representation derived from the chaos experienced (beta elements). Starting at the end and working backwards, my fear of abruptly interrupting the group could be linked to the children's frustrating experience a day earlier (and their fear) when they had expected us to have a group session; however, we had rushed off to go to another group (see chapter 8 for more details on this hypothesis).

3.2 Concluding remarks

This transcript vividly illustrates the importance of not getting lost in chaos. If one assumes that chaos means loss of control, one will not be able to contain it. Chaos should be perceived as a psychic state in which mental representations are lacking. Feelings of fear and anger are triggered by virtue of this absence of representation and are expressed intensely. Ensuring the presence of eclectic group conductors in the group setting, even in silence, is like providing a symbolic point of reference in the midst of chaos. We did adopt this approach in further chaotic situations in the group and it always worked pretty well.

4 Transcription 4: Fake family

Context: This transcription refers to the work of T-WAS at the end of the consolidation phase in shared housing for refugees for group S that took place weekly on Tuesdays from 5:30 to 7:00 pm. In total, the following children participated in the group that day: eight boys, Ra (aged 12), Sa (aged 11), Ab (aged 8), Di (aged 9), De (aged 11), Ta (aged 11), Am (aged 11) and Da (aged 8), and five girls, Pa (aged 9), Ne (aged 12), Del (aged 11), El (aged 10) and Deli (aged 8). As mentioned in previous chapters, this transcript refers to a time when the boys' and girls' groups from shared housing for refugees S started reflecting on having a mixed-gender group.

Progress: Due to traffic, we arrived five minutes late. De greeted us in the courtyard in the dark. Then, there were children in the corridor, some still working on their homework, with the help of some volunteers. Ta, a boy, gave a birthday gift to Leticia: 'Frozen' by Disney © magazine, with a lipstick toy and a make-up brush, costing 3.99 euros.

All for Leticia?

The volunteers said he had collected money from the other children so he could buy the gift. We quickly started to set up the chairs. Meanwhile, Leticia pretended to put on the make-up and the children laugh.

This is an extremely touching example of an 11-year-old boy organising himself – the boy in prepubescence expressing his emotions and his feelings of affection towards the female group conductor. The gift was accepted by Leticia when she pretended to put it on her face in front of the group. This gesture intentionally enabled her to show the gift to everyone and provided an appropriate tribute to it without shaming the boy.

Ra was also there, having often been absent this year. Right from the beginning, he was a loud character and he constantly wanted to be the centre of attention. Niko was immediately annoyed by him and took a deep breath, as whenever Niko wanted to say something, Ra interrupted him. As a result, Ra got two warnings in quick succession and Niko raised his voice while showing his annoyance.

From the social worker's perspective, we received information that his parents were currently separating and were constantly fighting, even in front of him. The presence of the police in the shared housing for refugees due to his parents' fights made the situation well-known across the whole camp.

Niko also tried to contain his aggressive energy by means proposed by Franck (1997).

The group began with the starting ritual. Leticia fought against Niko. Then, Leticia suggested splitting the group into two teams: girls versus boys. Niko advised that the leaders should choose the pairs. Leticia then gave one bataca bat to Ra and the other to Ne. Ne refused to play and wanted to leave the room. Niko moved quickly and playfully towards the door. She tried to push him away while other children tried to help her. Finally, she left the room. El, her sister, informed us that girls should not play with boys.

El's comment could be interpreted as 'girls should not have fun with boys after their menarche' – a very traditional cultural value. Being aware of her own biological development, Ne refused to play with Ra... It is true that Niko tried to encourage her by playing tag, but still, her cultural values were stronger.

Everyone else at this point accepted the respective matches and since there were more boys than girls, all the girls fought twice. Some girls stated they would like to play the sword fight (mashoonga).

Afterwards, we played cards and whilst playing, El and Pa whispered to Leticia that it was forbidden for them to sit on boys' laps for religious reasons. As the girls had played the bataca fight without complaining, we decided to consider their religious argument. Then, we arranged some long canes so that the children could be connected by holding the ends of them (see details in chapter 7).

The game was running smoothly. Some children hardly made any progress, but they were very patient. Di tried a few times to move around the circle, even though it was not his turn. Ta once slid backwards with his chair, so that almost everyone sitting on it fell down, and El and Ab won together. Niko went outside with them to find out what they wanted to play together next. Initially, both said they wanted to play Mashoonga, then El changed her decision to rubber chicken, and we did in fact have enough time for two games. Mashoonga was the first game. We let the two of them team up using rock-paper-scissors. The fight between Am and Deli was still quite childish – entirely defensive. Ra, at the end of the game, made everybody angry by saying that his team had won after all. 'But it's a tie', Leticia said.

Here, Leticia intended to give him back a reference point whilst reinforcing the energy invested by the 'losers'.

Meanwhile, the atmosphere grew heated and things got tense between Ra and Ta.

It was often unclear for us who started the physical fights, especially since for boys, it may be hard to admit that they were the first to be hit.

Following this, we played rubber chicken without the rubber chicken, as Niko had forgotten it. So, we replaced the rubber chicken with a plush turtle and a plastic spider. This worked quite well, too (see game details in chapter 7). On one occasion, Da cried because he had moved, and Ta tackled and blamed him, yet Da was not familiar with the game's rules. As there was still so much energy in the room, Leticia had the idea of playing a song for a dance-off. Niko started the music and played a popular song by Loredana, but the boys wanted a song by Sero and the girls started complaining, with comments going back and forth. While dancing, Ta accidentally punched Sa in his eye. Leticia quickly got a piece of frozen bread from the kitchen next door to cool it down (unfortunately, there were no ice packs).

Then Leticia came up with the idea of having two rows of children. The first child in one row would dance with the first child in the other row, and so on. Children were placed in lines at random. *The idea was to bring boys and girls together in a playful and harmless manner.*

When Ra once more messed up the game by refusing to dance together with little Deli (he was supposed to dance down the path with Deli, though he did this in front of her), Niko shouted several times 'together, together!' As a result, Niko showed in a loud voice that he was really fed up with Ra's disrespect towards the group. Even though a few children were overwhelmed by Niko's 'explosion', we kept playing, still having a lot of fun.

Niko tried to introduce a framework for Ra's aggressive energy by setting him boundaries as highlighted by Blom and Meier (2004), Oaklander (2001) and Bach and Goldberg (1976).

Farewell timeslot – thumbs-up/thumbs-down feedback: a few thumbs pointed down, a few up or in the middle. The mood was not the greatest. Di commented that he had also made mistakes; he knew that there had been a lot of arguing and he had also taken part in this. Pa thought that it had been incredibly loud, and Ra had been provoking others a lot. The two of them (Pa and Ra) bickered back and forth all the time, during which Ra really went into overdrive and mixed up many forms of devaluation: from ironic to spiteful laughter, mimicry and derogatory remarks about girls in general. Pa made him understand that he was being disrespectful. Niko pointed out that today was the third meeting, after which they would decide whether the girls wanted to play together with the boys. So far, things had gone well, but with Ra's presence, the session had changed a lot; there had been much more aggression in the room and fewer occasions when the children had actually played together. Niko saw no place for Ra in the group but wanted to discuss this with Leticia. From then on, Ra started openly saying that he would no longer be coming and asked everyone, one after the other, who wanted to join him. He came up with eight children who wanted to join him. Sa then said that although he would have football training on the same day as the group meeting, he would still come to the group.

Leticia and Niko pointed out that the group would start later, at 7 pm, from March onwards. Pa and El announced that they did not want to attend the group meeting any more. Leticia expressed her thoughts about Ra. She thought that at this moment, he was unable to enjoy being in the group, as he had a lot of anger and he directed it towards the group. He experienced these emotions and transferred them to the group, as we were a family. Then, Ra countered, 'What? Is this like a family? A fake family – that's what it is!'

Pa confirmed, 'Yes, we are like a family here. Even a fake family, but still a family!'

Leticia tried to keep talking to Ra and said that he (Ra) was empty, alone, afraid and angry – that is why he tried to break everything. He tried to keep provoking Leticia, but the resonance of Leticia's words brought calm to the group. Ra seemed to have lost his strength – it no longer resonated in the group.

Leticia used her mutuality skill combined with her maternal reverie mechanism by transforming into words the source of his anger. This was rarely adopted in the group setting as it is more of a typical interpretation. However, it is also a way of containing, which is how Niko had used it previously. Leticia sensed that the feelings of disintegration, emptiness, death, grief, loss, powerlessness were quite strong. The eclectic group conductors sensed the death that the children had witnessed in their lives during the group session.

We informed Ra that he would be allowed to return to the group only after we had had a one-on-one conversation with him. He was free to accept or reject this. Then, De made a joke, saying that he would come back next time because there would be a celebration of the month's birthdays. Niko took the joke further and ironically asked, 'What's that? Ah, cake, great!'

Niko's intention here was to highlight the polarity (divergence) between the emotional moment in group and the interruption on De's part.

Leticia emphasised that we would be there next week and anyone who would like to spend time with us would be more than welcome. Pa then said that she would come, but then again, it would depend on who else would be there. Ra wanted to leave; Leticia opened the door for him whilst telling him how sorry she was to see him go. He left without a word. The closing ritual was performed and goodbyes were said.

4.1 Eclectic group conductors' evaluation

Niko's thoughts: I find it problematic that the information about Ra's family situation was brought up abruptly by Leticia, even if this information was an 'open secret'. Nevertheless, the resonance triggered by Leticia's approach was quite interesting. Concerning the discussion about whether this group is a 'family' or not, this had, for the first time, been spoken about openly and urgently in the group.

Leticia's thoughts: The communication approach I had adopted with Ra was focused on TICA methods (Castrechini-Franieck, 2022) rather than on T-WAS approaches – an exception in children's group settings, as transference interpretations may inhibit the work of the group, as well as triggering the group's dependence on the group conductor (Woods 1996, p. 87). However, in this case, protecting the group setting from Ra's violence was imperative (Lehle 2018). To conclude, Ra came back to the group two weeks later and had agreed to talk to us in a two-to-one setting. He continued attending the group until our last meeting in March before the lockdown due to the COVID-19 pandemic (Niko's birthday celebration). From then on, we lost contact with him. However, the social workers said he had always been happy to receive our letters, even though we had not spoken to him since March.

As to the issue of whether the group was a 'fake family' or not, the different points of view were based on the children's different life experiences. Put more simply, Ra's reaction was quite reasonable, as at that time, he had just been experiencing the break-up of his family, whereas Pa's reaction was more than understandable as she had left her whole family behind when she was just six years old, to flee alone with one of her relatives to Germany.

4.2 Concluding remarks

This transcript includes 'penetrating situations', like in transcript 2, as well as a kind of 'rebellion' on the part of Ra. As in transcript 3, on one occasion, he tried to convince the other group members not to come to future group meetings. Nevertheless, as described in chapter 8, the dynamic group matrix of group S was characterised by the presence of strong resistance from the children with regards to playing freely in their neutral space, to trying to achieve homeostasis, and to aiming to achieve 'shared meaning communication'.

5 Some personal observations

Working with vulnerable children to prevent antisocial tendencies means being vulnerable to situations such as those described in this chapter – situations that can trigger past (and probably painful) memories or even put one's ability to surrender to the test. Because each group will have its own way of expressing aggression, there will be situations that cannot be predicted. It is important to be able to continue working in the midst of chaos, without 'being neither collapsing under that experience nor retaliating because of it' (Casement 1991, pp. 269–270).

References

Bach, G.R., and Goldberg, H., 1976. *Creative Aggression*. London: Coventure.

Ballhausen-Scharf, B., *et al.*, 2021. *Gruppenanalyse mit Kindern und Jugendlichen. Ein Leitfaden zur Kompetenzentwicklung*. Goettingen: Vandenhoeck & Ruprecht.

Bion, W.R., 1962. A theory of thinking. *International Journal of Psycho-Analysis*, 43, 4–5.

Bion, W.R., 1965. *Transformations: Change from Learning to Growth*. London: William Heinemann Medical Books.

Blom, H., and Meier, H., 2004. *Interkulturelles Management. Interkulturelle Kommunikation; internationales Personalmanagement; Diversity-Ansätze im Unternehmen*. 2nd ed. Herne: Verl. Neue Wirtschafts-Briefe.

Blom, R., 2006. *The Handbook of Gestalt Play Therapy: Practical Guidelines for Child Therapists*. London: Jessica Kingsley Publishers.

Casement, P., 1991. *Learning from the Patient*. New York, London: Guilford Press.

Cassorla, R.M.S., 2018. *The Psychoanalyst, the Theatre of Dreams and the Clinic of Enactment*. Abingdon, New York, NY: Routledge.

Castrechini-Franieck, L., ed., 2022. *Communication with Vulnerable Patients: A Novel Psychological Approach*. London: Routledge.

Foulkes, S.H., and Anthony, E.J., 1990. *Group Psychotherapy: The Psychoanalytic Approach*. 2nd ed. London: Routledge.

Franck, J., 1997. *Gestalt-Gruppentherapie mit Kindern*. 1st ed. Freiamt: Arbor-Verl.

Lehle, H.G., 2018. 'Egotraining in Aktion'. Das Spiel in der psychoanalytischen Kindergruppentherapie. In B. Traxl, ed. *Psychodynamik im Spiel. Psychoanalytische Überlegungen und klinische Erfahrungen zur Bedeutung des Spiels*. Frankfurt AM: Brandes & Apsel, 133–158.

Oaklander, V., 1988. *Windows to Our Children: A Gestalt Therapy Approach to Children and Adolescents*. Highland, NY: Center for Gestalt Development.

Oaklander, V., 2001. Gestalt play therapy. *International Journal of Play Therapy*, 10 (2), 45–55.

Winnicott, D.W., 1960. The theory of the parent-child relationship. *International Journal of Psycho-Analysis*, 41, 585–595.

Winnicott, D.W., *et al.*, eds., 2012/1984. *Deprivation and Delinquency*. Abingdon: Routledge.

Woods, J., 1996. Handling violence in child group therapy. *Group Analysis*, 29 (1), 81–98.

Chapter 10

Reflections on T-WAS (Together We Are Strong)

Throughout the book, the authors have shown how preventive psychosocial group work with children who are vulnerable (to prevent an increase in anti-social behaviour) can be achieved by means of T-WAS. Since several other people were also indirectly involved with the children (i.e., representatives of other children's services, social workers, etc.), it is definitely worth mentioning their thoughts about the visible improvement in the children's social behaviour while being involved in T-WAS. Therefore, most of this chapter reports their third party evaluation. This chapter also briefly outlines and classifies the general framework of T-WAS, including its content. Finally, T-WAS's limitations and potential are discussed.

1 Outcome of T-WAS from third parties[1]

This section presents a few items of feedback from third parties who have worked with the children on a regular basis.

1.1 Social workers from the shared housing for refugees where the groups took place

1.1.1 Team from shared housing for refugees S

We would like to thank you as a team for the successful children's group project in our accommodation, and we do this with one laughing eye and one crying eye.

Since the beginnings in July 2018, with separate boys' and girls' groups, to the last dates in December 2020 as a children's group (in which the latter gender had become secondary in terms of numbers), a lot has changed, and through close contact with us, we have always been involved in current developments or topics.

We would like to emphasise that both of you have overcome the hurdles that the pandemic has presented you with since the beginning of this year with great resourcefulness. Temporary visiting bans, limited group sizes in the

DOI: 10.4324/9781003466857-13

rooms, more difficult contact possibilities due to lack of telephone/internet resources etc., have complicated many things.

Therefore, we would like to thank you in particular for the fact that in times of the pandemic you 'stayed with' the children with great commitment and were the only reliable partner 'from outside' for a long period of time, who kept contact throughout and actively influenced the children's group experience.

1.1.2 Team from shared housing for refugees B

At present, 45 children and adolescents live in shared housing for refugees B (after the recent conversion to 7 m²); about 20 children belong to the target group of T-WAS. Unfortunately, we have had to observe above-average aggressive behaviour among the children in the past years, which is why an early connection to T-WAS was sought. Despite major efforts (reminders, accompanying the children to the group in shared housing for refugees T, parent talks, etc.), we did not succeed in making permanent contact with at least our 'most difficult' cases in the children's group in shared housing for refugees T, which is why we had already asked for an offer in B at the beginning of 2019.

After a long wait, Ms Franieck and Mr Bittner were finally able to start the children's groups we had long hoped for at the beginning of 2020. Right from the start, almost all the children of the corresponding age categories were present at the first group session. The feedback was extremely positive, and the children were very keen to continue. Then, COVID-19 regulations and the first lockdown put an abrupt end to this. With a lot of effort, Ms Franieck and Mr Bittner kept in touch with the children via WhatsApp and videos, riddles and phone calls and, as soon as it was possible, were on site again in-person. During lockdown, the TWAS children's group was a joyful change, and the transition to the 'real' group eventually went smoothly.

Based on the children's feedback, we have the impression that offering this group has been gratefully received. Even between the sessions, the children talk about and reflect on the processes, contents and dynamics of the group. Boundary violations become clear to the children, as does (in)appropriate aggressive behaviour from others and from themselves. Even at the few group events, the children already seem to gain a deeper understanding of the behaviour of all participants and increasingly begin to distinguish 'good' from 'bad' behaviour.

As professionals on site, we welcome the enormous commitment of Ms Franieck and Mr Bittner towards the children of shared housing for refugees B and are extremely curious to see how the children will develop in the course of the future. We consider the T-WAS children's group to be an irreplaceable service and are very grateful that it can take place here.

1.2 Guests from other organisations

1.2.1 Social worker, NGO

R. reported that after each group meeting, she felt extremely pleased with the activities and is flourishing properly. She is looking forward to the next one at the end of each session, which, in my opinion, encourages her in everyday life. She looks more confident and enjoys having a session with the group just for herself. With her nine siblings, she sometimes feels lost at home and is therefore all the more pleased about receiving the group's attention. It is very important that the group continues to meet regularly so that positive developments can be consolidated.

1.2.2 Art therapist, child protection centre

When I arrived in the shared housing for refugees, many children welcomed me in the group room. They waited excitedly until the group started at 5:30 pm. The mood was energetic and sometimes very turbulent. It was noticeable that the group was familiar with each other and had a sense of community. A reliable framework was created, in which the children could interact playfully with their peers and the consistent, adult caregivers (conductors). The children interacted in the social group and were able to learn that each personality has the right to be respected. Despite the daily obligations and the individual migration history, it would certainly be helpful for every single child to be able to take advantage of such support more often.

1.2.3 Mobile Youth Street Work

In the context of the project 'Power-Time' on the terrace of Mobile Youth Street Work, it happens time and again that young people who used to be in Leticia's children's group join us. These young people greeted Leticia joyfully and seemed surprised to meet her again together with us on the terrace of Mobile Youth Street Work (a well-known venue). Communication is much easier to establish thanks to the existing relationship that was built up through the children's group. The youths were able to talk about personal issues much sooner than the others, which facilitates the other youths in opening up more quickly in the group as well.

1.3 Review

As referred to in the preface, circa 70 children took part in T-WAS, yet some children came to us sporadically, while others were keen participants. Among the former are those youngsters who come these days to the project 'Power-Time' (see further details later in this chapter) on the terrace. However, they always ask about Niko and start bringing back lively and detailed memories of situations we experienced together in the children's group. Regarding the children who attended T-WAS regularly, these have achieved a stable state of emotional well-being while improving their behaviour at school and social skills.

2 Short overview and classification of T-WAS's general framework and its content

To enable the reader to classify the type of psychosocial group work outlined by T-WAS, the authors created a figure showing the relevant external and internal variables. Figure 10.1, therefore, classifies the basic framework and content orientation into ten variables, arranged according to a kind of point scale.

Psychosocial group work with children and its classification - Franieck and Bittner

Group goals	General ⟵————————————————————→ Specific
	Experience, general prevention Education Sensitisation Stabilisation Healing, therapy
Ways of thinking	Animation Motivation Learning Differentiation Experiential learning Personality development Self-awareness
Group types	Actions loose groups themes Ongoing social groups Social Group work Psychosocial group work Therapy group in addition to individual therapy
Typical places of use	Urban District Work Youth centre School Social/Educational Psychosocial Clinic private practices Street work Community Service Pre-school Organizations Institutions Sponsors Prison
Duration/ Frequency	Hours/days over months up to one year 1-2 years several years
Group sizes For face-to-face courses	Large group Class size Working group Small working group Small/therapy group 1:1 30+ 16-30 12-15 6-12 3-5
Leadership aspects	Structure-oriented ⟵————————→ Process-oriented
Group phases	0.5 years 1 year 1.5 years 2 years Group formation phase Consolidation phase Farewell phase
Composition	Different Mixed-sex Heterogeneous Multicultural Open Wide age range (biological/social) ⟷ Uniform Same-sex Homogeneous Monocultural Closed Small age range (biological/social)
Development issues	Collective ⟵————————————————→ Individual Group dynamics Communication/conflict management Community Trust Identity Meaning/values

Figure 10.1 Classification.

In terms of themes, the goals of the T-WAS focus on sensitisation and stabili-
sation, and the manner in which these goals are to be achieved is characterised
by experiential learning and self-development. As a type of psychosocial group
work, T-WAS has more overlaps with social group work than with therapy group
work and is more concerned with growth than with healing. In general, group
work in the social space is made up of collective social associations and it per-
forms a post-socialising function, which in this case meets the developmental
dynamics of children. Needless to say, the setting up of social group work should
be low-threshold, i.e., closer to home, in such a way as to provide easy access,
and being suitable for children (Slavson and Schiffer 1975, p. 429). Hence, the
work was conducted at the children's place of residence and was hosted by social
sponsors. Group lengths ranged from nine months to two and a half years, and
sessions were held weekly. Group sizes varied from a small class size to a small
working group, but if groups were gender separated, then they could mostly be
defined as small working groups. Initially, the focus of the group formation was
on a structure-oriented conductorship style. Progressively, the focus shifted to a
process orientation centred on the concept of eclectic group conductors. The
group composition tended to be more diverse and the emphasis on development
issues lay in community orientation.

3 Limitations

There are at least two emergent limitations at the relational level:

1   The resilience of group conductors. The most critical limitation
    of T-WAS is related to the 'wave of a psychotherapist's uncon-
    scious bias in their contact with "highly vulnerable/unbearable"
    patients or with deprived children, which is mostly triggered by
    transference and counter-transference issues' (Castrechini-Fra-
    nieck, 2022, p. 230). As highlighted in chapter 4, these biases
    require psychological resources that go far beyond the study of
    books. The dimension of self-regulation is constantly challenged
    when dealing with intense and archaic emotional charges in
    groups that do not yet have a representation. Or even the pre-
    sence of issues to be addressed that the group leaders may find
    difficult to deal with. Group leaders need to be able to deal with
    emotional stress. That's why we strongly recommend that group
    leaders, if they don't already have a personal training analysis
    (individual or group), have regular supervision. If this factor is
    neglected, the continuity of the group could be jeopardised. One
    or both group conductors may leave the group due to emotional
    overload. If only one of the group leaders stops leading the
    group and there is a replacement conductor, it will still be

possible to preserve the continuity of the group's development stages, despite this loss and mourning. Although this is not an ideal situation, because a process will be interrupted, losses are part of every life cycle. However, if there is no one to replace the outgoing group conductor, the end of the group should be communicated to the children well in advance, so that emotional support can be offered to help the group members cope with the abrupt interruption that is approaching.

2   Dealing with organisational dysfunction. If the staff of the facility (where the children's group meets) are not cooperative/supportive, do not understand the purpose of TWAS and do not ensure clear communication (for example, the room where the weekly group meets may be booked for another event, or may be full of furniture or decorated with objects that can be easily damaged), then the work of T-WAS will be negatively affected by these external influences. An additional challenge of crucial importance is certainly to make the staff of the organisation where the group takes place aware of the T-WAS goals. Another practical and critical factor is the duration of T-WAS (two years), which can be challenging for some organisations given the long-term funding required.

4 Some personal observations

As mentioned in chapter 8, the COVID-19 pandemic had a crucial impact on the work of T-WAS. Despite all our efforts to keep contact alive via films, we needed to abruptly interrupt our pair work as eclectic group conductors in December 2020. Since then, and as is expected (mainly based on the authors' foundation matrix), we, the eclectic group conductors, have been following separate paths in our work.

Since January 2021, Niko has also been working in 'open youth work' (OYW) again, in addition to school social work. The term 'open youth work' is defined in section 11 of Book VIII of the Social Code (SGB VIII) and is aimed at all young people, without any special criteria. OYW is located in a permanent building, such as a youth centre or a house, where young people may come voluntarily, without having to register, and they can take part in their activities on offer. OYW tends to provide open activities, i.e., recreational ones, educational ones, courses, projects, etc. Community work is aimed at individual young people or cliques/groups of friends and includes leisure activities, as well as educational or counselling services in the transition from school to work. Working with a female colleague, Niko has retained the basic structure of eclectic group conductors in his work. The creative games used in T-WAS are also still in his repertoire, with a focus on tapping into ego-strengthening and family-like experiences.

Since September 2021, Leticia has been working in partnership with 'mobile young street work' (MYSW) following the rampage on the streets of Stuttgart in June 2020. 'Mobile Youth Street Work' is linked to section 13 SGB VIII and has a clearly defined target group, namely people aged 14–27, who are threatened or affected by social deprivation and who are not or not adequately covered by other youth work, youth social work or youth welfare services. In terms of methodology, MYSW works with four pillars: street work, one-to-one help, group work and community work. In addition, it aims to be on the street. MYSW is conducted in various places where young people can be found, such as on the street or in public places. The idea is to collect young people from their current location and offer them support in coping with individual and structural living conditions.

In Leticia's work, she has been trying to minimise the aggressive behaviour of young people by means of establishing a human relationship of trust. In this setting, it is possible to offer the youngsters a neutral, safe and available space, to which they can turn when they are emotionally challenged. To achieve this, Leticia has adopted and adapted a combination of approaches from TICA and T-WAS. In particular, she has still been working with the concept of eclectic group conductors, but owing to the circumstances at the setting, her partner is no longer a single person, but rather a team – the street work team. In addition, since March 2023, Leticia has resumed her work with T-WAS and has kept the basic structure of the eclectic group conductors. Once again in two different types of shared accommodation for refugees.

The different career paths of the authors clearly illustrate how T-WAS can be implemented and adapted in different settings and particular circumstances. This makes it an eminently suitable approach or tool for group psychosocial work with vulnerable children and young people.

Note

1 From chapter 10, pp. 217–219, *Communicating with Vulnerable Patients: A Novel Psychological Approach*, by Maria Leticia Castrechini Fernandes Franieck, © 2023 by Imprint. Reproduced by Routledge, permission of Taylor & Francis Group.

References

Castrechini-Franieck, L., ed., 2022. *Communication with Vulnerable Patients: A Novel Psychological Approach*. London: Routledge.
Slavson, S.R., and Schiffer, M., 1975. *Group Psychotherapies for Children: A Textbook*. New York: International Universities Press.

Index

Bold page numbers indicate tables, *italic* numbers indicate figures.

aggression: challenges from children 100–118; expression of anger 10; facets of 8–10; primary 11, suppression of 09; processing of in group work 11–12; shared meaning communication 12; shift from punishment to treatment x

aggressive energy: batacas 'fights' 58–61; children in Gestalt therapy 16; inward/outward turned 16–17; release through playfulness 53; rules of the group and 47

anger, expression of 10

anger management: batacas 'fights' 58–61; belt-pulling fights 63–64; boxing with/without punching bags 64–65; creative group play 58–67, *66*; Haka game 67; mashoonga fights 62–63; non-ritualised 62–67, *66*, 80; as pillar of T-WAS 50, *51*; primal screams 61–62; ritualised 58–62; throwing games with balls 65–66, *66*; water fights 66–67

Anthony, E.J. 12, 13, 25–26, 28, 45, 50, 59

anti-social tendencies: and anti-social acts 7–8; group work and 11–13; primary aggression, suppression of 11; Winnicott on 7–8

art therapist's evaluation of T-WAS 121

authors, foundation matrix of 35–38

Bach, G.R. 10

Ballhausen-Scharf, B. 26–27, 29

batacas 'fights' 53, 58–61

Bauer, J. 9

being glued to the wall game 69

belt-pulling fights 63–64

biological facet of aggression 9

Bion, W.R. 11, 18, 20–21, 26, 55, 59, 73

birthday celebrations 75

Bittner, N. 12, 40–41; foundation matrix of 36–38

blind cow game 72

Blom, R. 10, 17, 55

Bonaparte, M. xi

boundaries: reasons for setting 10; setting 55

boxing with/without punching bags 64–65

Brandes, H. 26

burn ball 65, *66*

card game 53, 67–68

carrot pulling game 72–73

Casriel, D. 10

Castrechini-Franieck, L. 1, 12, 19, 40–41; foundation matrix of 35–36, 38

chaos xvi, 73, 109; psychological chaos 111–113; 118

children in Gestalt therapy 16–18

Cividini-Strani, E. 28

closing rituals for meetings 53–54, 56, 61–62

co-leadership of groups 28–29, 30; *see also* eclectic group conductors; leadership in group work

communication *see* shared meaning communication

conductors, group leaders as 26, 28; *see also* eclectic group conductors

conflicts, handling of 44–45, 100–118

consolidation phase 52

contact functions, training of 17

container-contained interaction 20, 21, 44, 73, 88
cooking 74
COVID-19: contact design during 79–80, 81–82, **83–86**, 89; refugee shared housing, groups run in 96–98
creative group play: anger management 58–67, *66*; batacas 'fights' 58–61; being glued to the wall game 69; belt-pulling fights 63–64; birthday celebrations 75; blind cow game 72; boxing with/without punching bags 64–65; card game 67–68; carrot pulling game 72–73; celebration of birthdays 75; cooking 74; dancing 73–74; dream bags 77; ego-strengthening 67–78, *70*; excrement machine 77–78; excursions 76; family-like experiences 73–77; film evenings 76; Haka game 67; imagination, encouragement of 77–78; interpretation of games 80; mashoonga fights 62–63; musical chairs game 71–72; musical statues game 72; non-ritualised anger management 62–67, *66*; painting projects 75–76; photo projects 76–77; physical exercises 74–75; primal screams 61–62; reflection 78; ritualised anger management 58–61; rubber chicken game 69–71, *70*; singing 73; social togetherness, promotion of 67–73, *70*; throwing games with balls 65–66, *66*; thumbprint 78; transcriptions 78; in T-WAS 2; water fights 66–67

dilemma (reflects polarity) 40–41, 53, 94, 99, 104
Diploma in Forensic Psychotherapy xii
diversity, attitude towards 48
dodgeball 65–66
dream bags 77
dream work 20–21

eclectic group conductors: aggressive challenges from children 100–118; authors' foundation matrixes and 38; conflict handling 44–45, 100–118; diversity, attitude towards 48; group structure, maintenance of 47–48; introducing 41; miscommunication example 101–103; mutual understanding communication 43–44; parental representation, awareness of role 45; as pillar of T-WAS *51*; play

skills 45–46, *46*; procedures 43–45; professional exchange 44; resilience of 123–124; roles 42–43; rule checks 47–48; shared meaning communication 40; supervision 45; in T-WAS 2; as unit or individuals 41–42, *42*; variables influencing 42, *43*
ego-relatedness 2, 12 ego-relatedness frame 8, 12
ego-strengthening: being glued to the wall game 69; birthday celebrations 75; blind cow game 72; card game 67–68; carrot pulling game 72–73; celebration of birthdays 75; cooking 74; creative group play 67–78, *70*; dancing 73–74; dream bags 77; excrement machine 77–78; excursions 76; family-like experiences 73–77; film evenings 76; imagination, encouragement of 77–78; musical chairs game 71–72; musical statues game 72; painting projects 75–76; photo projects 76–77; physical exercises 74–75; as pillar of T-WAS 50, *51*; rubber chicken game 69–71, *70*; singing 73
emotional containment 26
emotional settling in of leaders 43–44
epistemic-psychoanalytic perspective leadership in group work 25–26
excrement machine 77–78
excursions 76, 93
experiential knowledge 18
external objects, emotional communication facilitation and 1

facilities where groups meet 124
family-like relationship 29
family-like experiences in creative group play: birthday celebrations 75; cooking 74; dancing 73–74; excursions 76; fake family 113–117; film evenings 76; painting projects 75–76; photo projects 76–77; physical exercises 74–75; singing 73
farewell phase 52–53
farewell timeslot 53–54
film evenings 76
forensic psychotherapy: formalization xii; origins x–xi
formation phase of groups 52, 88–89
Foulkes, E. 12–13

Foulkes, S.H. 12–13, 26, 28, 45, 50, 55, 56, 59
foundation matrix: authors' 35–38; defined 13
Franck, J. 24, 25
Freud, S. 18, x–xi

gender: co-leadership of groups and 28–29; refugee shared housing, groups run in 90, 91, 95–96, 98, 103–108; role swapping 77
Gestalt therapy: children in 16–18; homeostasis 11, 16; ontological psychoanalysis and 21–22
Gilligan, J. 8
Ginott, H.G. 55
Goldberg, H. 10
group conductors: conductors, group leaders as 26; foundation matrix of 35–38; see also eclectic group conductors
group dynamic matrix 13
group foundation matrix 13, 35–38
group personal matrix 13, 38
group formation phase 52, 88–89
group leadership see leadership in group work
group matrix 12–13, 27
groups: aggression, processing of in 11–12; features of 29; powers of xv; structure of, maintenance of 47–48; see also eclectic group conductors; leadership in group work

Haar, R. 28
Hacker, F. 8
Haka game 67
Hofmann, E. 26
holding 19–20, 26, 27
homeostasis in Gestalt therapy 11, 16

imagination, encouragement of 77–78
International Association for Forensic Psychotherapy xii

James, D.C. 12

Kirsch, C. 28
Klain, E. 28
Klein, M. 18, xi

leadership in group work: aggressive energy, expressions of and 25; co-leadership 28–29, 30; conductors, leaders as 26; disruptions, handling 29; epistemic-psychoanalytic perspective 25–26; models of group work and 24–27; ontological-psychoanalytic perspective 26–27, 29; role of the leader(s) 24–27, 29; violent impulses, toleration and transformation of 58; see also eclectic group conductors
Lehle, H.G. 26–27, 55
length of group 52
Lucas, T. 12, 27, 58

Mann, D. 9
mashoonga fights 62–63
maternal reverie 20, 21, 27, 45, 73
methodological pillars of T-WAS 50, 51, 52
miscommunication by eclectic group conductors (example) 101–103
Mobile Youth Street Work: evaluation of T-WAS 121; target groups and methodology 125
Moll, M. 27, 29
moments of meeting 19, 27
musical chairs game 71–72
musical statues game 72
mutuality, process of 19, 44, 88
mutual understanding communication 43–44

non-ritualised anger management: belt-pulling fights 63–64; boxing with/ without punching bags 64–65; Haka game 67; introduction of games 80; mashoonga fights 62–63; throwing games with balls 65–66, 66; water fights 66–67

Oaklander, V. 9, 24, 59–60
Ogden, T.H. 18, 19, 20
ontological psychoanalysis: communication by 18–21; Gestalt therapy and 21–22; leadership in group work and 26–27, 29
open nature of groups 54, 56
open youth work 124
organisations where groups meet 124
organismic self-regulation 16–18
Other, the, maintaining contact with 35

'Paarleitung', use of term in Germany 29
painting projects 75–76
pair leadership of groups *see* eclectic
   group conductors; leadership in group
   work
parental representation, awareness of
   role 45
Perls, F.S. 9
personal matrix 13; authors' 38
phases of T-WAS 52–53, 56
photo projects 76–77
physical exercises 74–75
pillars, methodological, of T-WAS 50,
   51, 52
play: children in Gestalt therapy 16–18;
   ritualised/non-ritualised 50; skills of
   eclectic group conductors 45–46, *46*;
   see also creative group play
playtime timeslot 53
poo machine 77–78
positive facet of aggression 9–10
powers of groups xv
primal screams 54, 61–62
primary aggression: shared meaning
   communication 12; suppression of 11
professional exchange 44
psychoanalysis, value of in criminality
   studies xi

Rahm, D. 28
reflection: as pillar of T-WAS 50, *51*, 52;
   thumbprint 78; transcriptions 78
refugee children 40
refugee shared housing, groups run in: B
   group 89, 97–98, 120; conflict in 92, *92*,
   96; considerate attitude of children 90;
   COVID-19 and 96–98; ending of
   groups 93, 96; ethnic conflicts 89;
   excursion 93; (fake) family, groups as
   113–117; formation phase of groups
   88–89; gender and 90, 91, 95–96, 98,
   103–108; painting project 93; parallels
   between groups *89*, 89–90; rebellion in
   a group 109–113; rules of the group 93;
   S group 88–89, 94–97, 119–120; shared
   meaning communication 91, 93, 95;
   sports programme in competition with
   94–95; T group 88, 90–93, *92*, *94*
relational representations 27
resilience: of eclectic group conductors
   123–124; Gestalt therapy as
   promoting 17

ritualised anger management: batacas
   'fights' 58–61; primal screams 61–62
ritualised/non-ritualised play 50
rubber chicken game 69–71, *70*
rule checks 47–48

Sachs, H. xi
self-regulation, children in Gestalt
   therapy and 16–18
shame, violence and 8–9
shared implicit relationship 18
shared meaning communication xvi;
   eclectic group conductors 40–41;
   primary aggression, acknowledgment
   of 12; refugee shared housing, groups
   run in 91, 93, 95; in T-WAS 2
singing 73
Slavson, S.R. 25, 28
social facet of aggression 9
social togetherness, promotion of: being
   glued to the wall game 69; blind cow
   game 72; card game 67–68; carrot
   pulling game 72–73; musical chairs
   game 71–72; musical statues game 72;
   rubber chicken game 69–71, *70*
social workers' evaluations of T-WAS
   119–121
starting ritual 58–61
Stern, D.N. 18, 27
structure of the group, maintenance of
   47–48
supervision 45

thinking 'either-or' vs. 'both-as-also'
   40–41, 53, 102–103
throwing games with balls 65–66, *66*
thumbprint 78
TICA (Transient Interactive
   Communication Approach) 1
timescale of groups 52
time structure of meetings 53–54, 56
'Together We Are Strong' *see* T-WAS
   (Together We Are Strong)
transcriptions 78
Transient Interactive Communication
   Approach (TICA) 1
transitional phenomena (also transitional
   space) 13, 19–20, 26, 27
Trautmann-Voigt, S. 28
T-WAS (Together We Are Strong): aims
   xv; anger management 50, *51*;
   authors' foundation matrixes and 38;

boundary setting 55; COVID-19
and 79–80, 81–82, **83–86**, 89;
ego-strengthening 50, *51*; facilities for
meetings 124; formation of group in
refugee housing 54–55; limitations
123–124; with Mobile Youth Street
Work 125; open nature of groups 54,
56; overview 123; phases of 52–53, 56;
pillars, methodological 50, *51*, 52;
powers of groups xv; reflection 50, *51*,
52; ritualised/non-ritualised play 50;
shared meaning communication 2; size
of groups 54, 56; starting point for 7;
third party evaluations of 119–122;
TICA and 1; timescale of groups 52;
time structure of meetings 53–54,
56; variables *122*; videos about
development of **3**, 4; *see also* eclectic
group conductors; leadership in group
work; refugee shared housing,
groups run in

violence as facet of aggression 8–9
Voigt, B. 28

water fights 66–67
welcome timeslot 53
Welldon, E.V. xii
Wenzel, H. 28
Westman, A. 29, 42
Westwick, A. xi
Wheeler, G. 11
Williams, A. 18–19
Winnicott, D.W. 2, 7–8, 9, 11, 13, 18, 19, 20
Wirth, W. 24
Woods, J. 11, 27, 55

zombie dodgeball 65–66

For Product Safety Concerns and Information please contact our EU
representative GPSR@taylorandfrancis.com Taylor & Francis Verlag GmbH,
Kaufingerstraße 24, 80331 München, Germany

Printed and bound by CPI Group (UK) Ltd, Croydon, CR0 4YY

08/06/2025

01897006-0015